I0421781

# Who Cares?

*Your Essential Guide to Aged Care in Australia*

All rights reserved. No part of this publication may be reproduced, stored in a retrieval system or transmitted in any form by any means, electronic, mechanical, photocopying, recorded or otherwise, without the prior written permission of the copyright owner.

ISBN 978-0-6456862-9-6

Published by Sunday Press Melbourne
Copyright © Sunday Press Melbourne
Designed & Written by Jonette George
jonette@sundaypress.com.au

The material in this publication is of the nature of general comment only, and does not represent professional advice. It is not intended to provide specific guidance for particular circumstances and it should not be relied on as the basis for any decision to take action or not take action on any matter it covers. Readers should obtain professional advice where appropriate, before making any such decision. To the maximum extent permitted by law, the author and publishers disclaim all responsibility and liability to any person, arising directly or indirectly from any person taking or not taking action based on the information in this publication.

# Who Cares?

## Your Essential Guide to Aged Care in Australia

Jonette George

# TABLE OF CONTENTS

# *INTRODUCTION*

I wrote this book from my experience caring for my elderly parents and cousin while navigating the aged care system. It is designed to help you and your family avoid some of the pitfalls we encountered along the way.

## *KEY STATISTICS REGARDING FAMILY AGED CARE*

### TOTAL INFORMAL CARERS
Around 3 million Australians provide unpaid care,
which includes care for the frail aged.

### FAMILY AS PRIMARY CARERS
Approximately 96% of primary carers
(the person providing the most care) look after a family member.

### NUMBER OF PRIMARY CARERS
There are roughly 1.2 million primary carers in Australia.

### CARING FOR OLDER PEOPLE
Around 35.3% of Australia's family and friend carers
look after someone over the age of 65.

(Australian Institute of Health and Welfare)

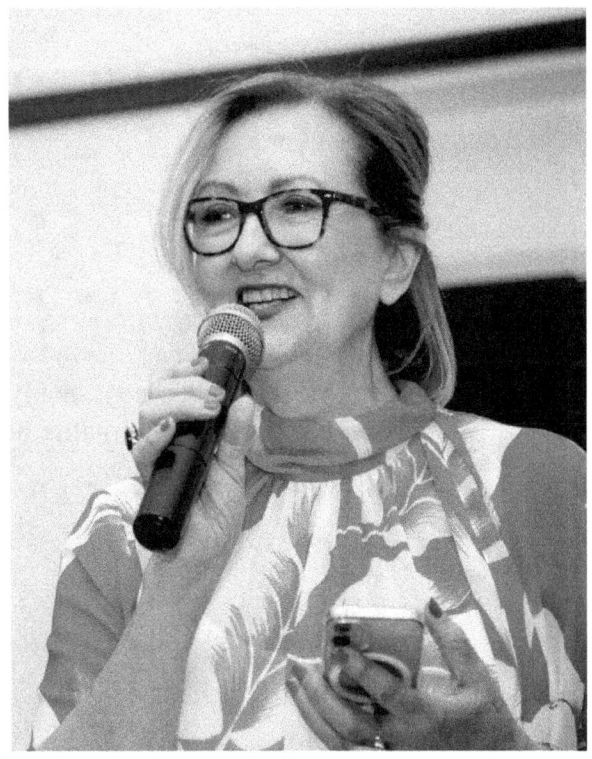

Jonette George is a dynamic and passionate figure in the Australian publishing industry, with more than 25 years' experience producing practical, plain-language guides. She is known for conducting in-depth research and interviews, translating complex systems into clear explanations, and providing readers with confident, actionable guidance.

At the beginning of the COVID-19 pandemic, Jonette moved to Noosa to care for her ageing parents. Over the following five years, she experienced both the best and the worst of Australia's aged care, health, and legal systems — experiences that led her to write Who Cares? in the hope of sparing other families the confusion, stress, and trauma she encountered.

Jonette's understanding of aged care deepened further through her role supporting her cousin during serious illness. This period exposed her to the realities of fluctuating capacity, contested decision-making, breakdowns in communication between services, and the emotional toll placed on families when medical, legal, and care systems fail to work together. Earlier, Jonette's father — a retired GP — entered an aged care home for a planned two-week respite while she travelled to Melbourne to meet her new grandson.

On the eighth day, after receiving concerning reports from his regular carers, speaking with a dismissive clinical staff member at the facility, and hearing her father wheezing and coughing over the phone, Jonette flew home and took him straight to hospital.

He was admitted with malnutrition and spent a week being hand-fed to reverse what his physician described as a near-palliative situation.

How can things go so wrong in such a short space of time?

Jonette believes that being informed about the rights of older people — and understanding how health, aged care, and legal frameworks intersect — is one of the most powerful tools families have. Knowing what questions to ask, and when to ask them, helps cut through bureaucracy and puts care providers on notice that indifference, neglect, and poor communication will not be accepted.

# WHY I WROTE THIS BOOK

I left Melbourne during the pandemic, at the very start of lock downs - in fact, the day before the gates were locked. I packed a small suitcase, thinking my trip would be a matter of weeks, to look after my elderly parents.

My father would turn 90 the day after my arrival, and my mother turned 90 later that year.

I am still here in Noosa, six years later.

Inadvertently, I had signed up for their rest-of-life journey, but at the time, I thought I was keeping the evil pandemic from their doors.

What I have learnt over the last six years is worth bottling, and I just wish I knew as much at the start of the journey as what I do now.

I have written this book as a guide to anyone who has elderly parents and wishes to support them through their last years. It is an honourable journey but it is fraught with mistakes, emotion, anguish and pain - both for your parents and for yourself.

The aged care system in Australia is complex and it would be very difficult to navigate if you didn't have someone to guide you.

My mother has since passed away, but her last words on her death bed were telling my daughter how wonderful Jonette has been. She repeatedly claimed, "She has given me dignity."

*"If I didn't have a daughter,*
*where would I be today?*
*Over the hills and far away*
*from loved ones young and old*
*but only a daughter can be so bold*
*to stand up for me, good as gold.*

*Over her body to a strange land*
*so my sacred home could be sold.*
*I've spent years, fighting for my rights*
*I claim no shame, I'm only a name.*

*But my daughter ensures my dignity*
*protecting me from all signatories*
*signing my rights away.*

*So the old saying,*
*Fake it 'til you make it*
*has been my creed in need*
*because my daughter will make sure*
*I make it."*

Dec 19, 2021.
Merveen George

I just wish I understood the systems better to improve my mother's final years, but I did my best.

And with my father, who passed away aged 95, I did my best.

We worked our way through the system, getting him on a Level 4 package so he could stay at home.

I organised the care he needed to make that possibility a reality and, as his world shrunk between his bed and chair in front of the TV, he was grateful that he could live out his life the way he hoped.

Despite forays into hospitals for various ailments, and a very unfortunate week in respite care in a local nursing home, we did well. Again, if I knew the questions one should ask a nursing home, his respite (and my little holiday to visit my first grandchild) wouldn't have turned out the way it did.

After eight days of "care", Dad was admitted to Noosa Hospital for malnutrition - he had an extraordinary weight loss in eight days. They simply had no supervision over his nutrition and his meals slipped by the wayside.

The Aged Care Quality and Safety Commission investigated and after twelve months of rigorous testing, found four major GAPS in the home's procedures, and after writing a report filled with recommendations, the Aged Care Facility was made to rectify them so they wouldn't hurt anyone else.

Then I received a frantic call from my cousin, who had end-stage kidney failure. She asked me to come as soon as possible to care for her during what she believed would be her final days. I did not hesitate. She said her regular carer had left and could not return. She said she needed help.

I left my family ski trip early and flew to her regional city within a few days. I ended up staying for four months. During that time I encountered another set of failures — this time the quiet sidelining and ghosting of the family carer.

Despite severe confusion from advanced uraemia, episodes of delusion — including telling health professionals I was trying to kill her by withholding food — and clear signs of progressing dementia, she was assessed as safe to live at home alone, at least until the next hospital admission.

Eventually it became clear that the system was not going to recognise what was happening.

That moment changed everything for me.

I wrote this guide so that no other family has to face such chaotic and frightening end-of-life decisions without understanding the system around them.

*Jonette George*

# *HOW TO USE THIS BOOK*

This guide follows the typical journey carers experience when supporting an older person through the aged care system.

You do not need to read it strictly from beginning to end.

**If you are early in the journey, start with:**
- Chapter 3 – How the System Really Works
- Chapter 5 – Assessments Without Tears

**If you are navigating services at home:**
- Chapter 9 – Money, Payments and the Myth of Support
- Chapter 10 – Care at Home

**If you are considering residential care:**
Chapter 14 – Choosing an Aged Care Facility

**If your family member is approaching end of life:**
Chapter X – End-of-Life and Palliative Care

**If caring has recently ended:**
Chapter 17 – After Caring

Each chapter ends with a short section titled What This Chapter Wants You to Know to help summarise the key points.

# UNDERSTANDING THE AGED CARE SYSTEM
# IN AUSTRALIA

## A SIMPLE SYSTEM MAP FOR CARERS

The aged care system can feel complex when you first enter it. There are multiple agencies, assessments and funding programs. Understanding how the pieces fit together helps carers navigate the process more confidently and avoid delays.

The structure below shows how most people move through the system.

## PUTTING THE SYSTEM TOGETHER

A simplified pathway through the aged care system usually follows this sequence:

**Step 1**
Contact My Aged Care

**Step 2**
Assessment by RAS or ACAT

**Step 3**
Eligibility for government-funded services

**Step 4**
Support delivered at home through Support at Home programs
or
Transition into residential aged care

**Step 5**
Oversight from regulators and legal bodies if needed

## HOW RESIDENTIAL AGED CARE COSTS WORK

When entering residential aged care, residents may be asked to contribute to accommodation costs. These can be paid as a lump sum (RAD), a daily payment (DAP) or a combination of both. Government means testing determines whether additional care fees apply based on income and assets.

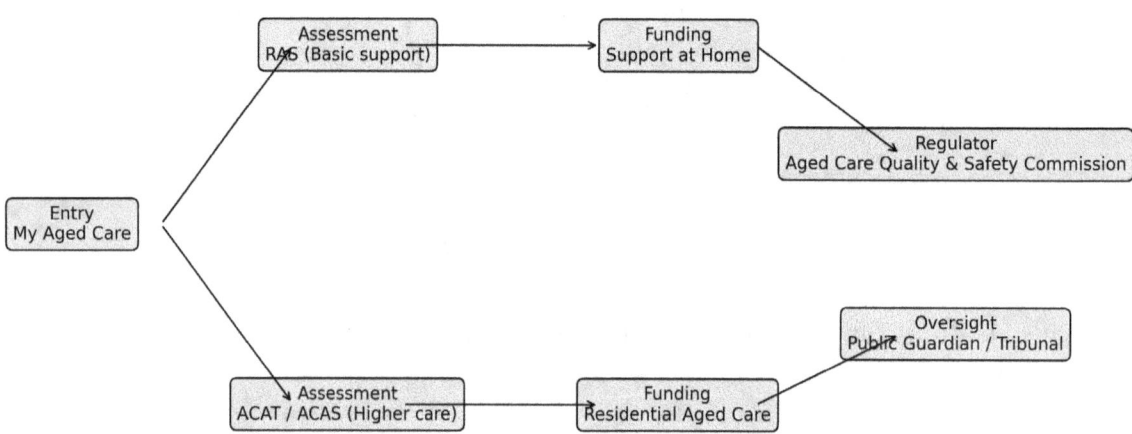

## WHY UNDERSTANDING THE SYSTEM MATTERS

The aged care system involves multiple agencies and decision points. Carers who understand how the system is structured are better able to:

request the right assessments

challenge unsafe decisions

escalate concerns when care is inadequate

access the services their family member is entitled to receive

While the system can appear bureaucratic, knowing the pathway helps carers navigate it more effectively and advocate with confidence.

## THE SYSTEM IN BRIEF

### 1. Entry Point
**My Aged Care**
For most Australians, the journey into aged care begins with My Aged Care, the Australian Government's central access point for aged care services.

My Aged Care provides:
- information about available services
- eligibility screening
- referrals for assessment
- a national database of service providers

Families can contact My Aged Care online or by phone. Information collected during this first contact includes:
- personal details
- health concerns
- mobility issues
- support currently provided by family or carers
- safety risks in the home

Based on this initial conversation, My Aged Care refers the person for a formal assessment.


## 2. Assessment Pathways
There are two different assessment teams depending on the level of care needed.
- RAS – Regional Assessment Service
- RAS assessments are used for lower-level support needs.

They determine eligibility for services under the Commonwealth Home Support Programme (CHSP) and similar entry-level support programs.

## RAS ASSESSMENTS
A RAS assessor usually visits the person at home and evaluates:
- daily living needs
- home safety
- mobility and independence
- social support
- carer capacity

RAS assessments focus on maintaining independence and delaying the need for more intensive care. Typical services approved after a RAS assessment may include:
- cleaning and domestic help
- meal services
- transport
- social support
- minor home maintenance

## ACAT / ACAS – AGED CARE ASSESSMENT TEAM / SERVICE

ACAT (called ACAS in Victoria) assessments are required for higher-level aged care services. These include:

- Home Care Packages
- residential aged care
- residential respite care
- transition care after hospital

The assessment team usually includes health professionals such as nurses, doctors or social workers. They assess:

- medical needs
- cognitive capacity
- mobility and safety
- ability to live independently
- carer support and sustainability

The ACAT assessment determines what level of government-funded care the person is eligible to receive.

### 3. Funding Streams

Once eligibility is confirmed, funding can be allocated through one of the main aged care programs.

### Support at Home

The Support at Home program is a major reform replacing the previous Home Care Package and Commonwealth Home Support programs.

Its aim is to provide a simpler system for supporting older people living at home. Funding can cover services such as:

- personal care
- nursing support
- physiotherapy and allied health
- domestic assistance
- home modifications
- assistive equipment

The goal of Support at Home is to help people remain living safely in their own home for as long as possible.

**Residential Aged Care Funding**
When living at home is no longer safe or sustainable, people may move into residential aged care. Residential care provides:
- accommodation
- 24-hour care
- nursing support
- meals and daily living assistance
- access to allied health services

Funding for residential care typically involves a combination of:
- government subsidy
- resident contributions
- accommodation payments

These payments may include:
- a Refundable Accommodation Deposit (RAD)
- a Daily Accommodation Payment (DAP)
- means-tested care fees depending on financial circumstances

**4. Regulation**
**Aged Care Quality and Safety Commission**
The Aged Care Quality and Safety Commission is the national regulator responsible for overseeing aged care providers. Its responsibilities include:
- monitoring provider compliance with quality standards
- investigating complaints from residents, families and carers
- auditing aged care services
- enforcing safety and quality requirements
- overseeing incident reporting under the Serious Incident Response Scheme

If families believe a provider is not meeting expected standards of care, complaints can be lodged with the Commission.

## 5. Oversight and Legal Safeguards

Sometimes older people lose the ability to make decisions about their own care, finances or living arrangements. When this occurs, oversight mechanisms may become involved.

### Public Guardian or Public Advocate

State-based offices that protect the rights of people who lack decision-making capacity.

They may be appointed to make decisions about:
- medical treatment
- living arrangements
- personal welfare

### Civil and Administrative Tribunals

Each state has a tribunal that can appoint:
- guardians for personal decisions
- administrators for financial matters

Tribunals are usually involved when:
- there is family disagreement
- no enduring power of attorney exists
- someone is being financially exploited
- the person is unable to make decisions safely

Tribunals provide legal oversight to ensure decisions are made in the person's best interests.

# Chapter 1

## *DON'T DO IT!*
### *(UNLESS YOU LOVE SOMEONE THAT MUCH)*

If you're reading this because you're thinking about becoming a carer, let me be very clear from the outset:

Don't do it!
Put this book down!
Back away slowly!
Go and live your life while you still can!

And if you're already a carer—well, I'm sorry. It's too late now. You're one of us.

Because nobody chooses this job in the traditional sense. You don't apply for it on Seek. There's no interview panel, no probation period, no polite email saying, "Thank you for your application, but we've decided to go with someone else." Instead, you're drafted. Conscripted. Thrown into the deep end without floaties, without training, and very often without warning.

One day you're a daughter, a spouse, a son, a sibling, a partner. The next day you're managing medications, bodily fluids, emotional meltdowns, medical appointments, Centrelink forms, and the slow, aching grief of watching someone you love disappear in front of you.

### *WELCOME TO CAREGIVING.*

## HOW WE END UP HERE - WHETHER WE LIKE IT OR NOT

No one sits around the dinner table and says, "You know what I'd love to do in my forties, fifties, or seventies? Give up my income, my freedom, my privacy, and most of my sanity to become a full-time unpaid nurse."

Yet here we are.

Sometimes it starts quietly. A missed appointment. Burnt toast. Repeating the same story three times in one conversation. A fall. A diagnosis that lands like a punch to the chest.

Sometimes it's sudden. A stroke. An accident. A hospital discharge that comes with the terrifying words: "They can't live alone anymore."

And sometimes—cruelly—it sneaks up on you so slowly that you don't realise when your life stopped being yours.

You don't become a carer in one big moment.

You slide into it.

One favour. One night stay. One "just for a few weeks."

Until suddenly you are it.

And everyone else assumes you'll cope. Because you always have.

## THE MYTH OF THE CARER'S PAYMENT

Let's talk about the elephant in the room: the money.

Yes, there is a Carer Payment.

Yes, it's around $500 a week.

No, that does not make this job easy, fair, or adequately compensated.

That payment doesn't cover:

- The lost superannuation
- The stalled career
- The isolation
- The exhaustion
- The emotional labour
- The nights you lie awake listening for movement
- The days you don't get to shower
- The years shaved off your own health

It certainly doesn't cover the fact that you are on duty 24 hours a day, often without weekends, sick leave, or holidays.

If caregiving were paid at award rates—factoring in nursing, personal care, emotional support, administration, cleaning, cooking, and crisis management—you'd be on six figures.

Instead, you get a fortnightly payment and a quiet expectation that love will fill the gaps.

Spoiler alert: love helps—but it doesn't stop burnout.

# *LET'S NOT SUGARCOAT THIS: IT IS HARD*

Caregiving is not Instagram-worthy.

It is not matching scrubs and smiling selfies.

It is dementia, where the person you love looks at you with suspicion, fear or anger because your face no longer registers as familiar.

It is incontinence, where dignity becomes a daily negotiation and bodily functions take centre stage in ways you never imagined.

It is lifting, cleaning, washing, changing, coaxing, pleading and sometimes crying in the laundry because it's the only quiet place left.

It is repeating the same answer forty times a day.

It is being accused of stealing, lying, or plotting — by the very person you are sacrificing everything for.

It is medical appointments that run late, doctors who speak in acronyms, and systems that assume you have infinite energy and infinite patience.

It is grief layered on top of grief — because the person is still here, but also not.

And no one really prepares you for that.

## *DEMENTIA: LOVING SOMEONE WHO IS LEAVING*

Dementia deserves its own warning label.

- It is not just memory loss.
- It is personality loss.
- It is role reversal on steroids.

You become the parent. The decision-maker. The keeper of reality.

You grieve in instalments. Every lost skill. Every forgotten name. Every moment of clarity that fades again.

And yet—you still love them. Fiercely. Stubbornly. Exhaustedly.

You love them when they don't know who you are.

You love them when they lash out.

You love them when they beg to "go home," even though they're already there.

That kind of love is not for the faint-hearted.

# INCONTINENCE

## THE TABOO NOBODY WARNS YOU ABOUT

No one talks about this enough, so let's do it properly.

- Incontinence is confronting.
- It strips away modesty—yours and theirs.
- It forces intimacy you never expected to share.

There are smells. Accidents. Middle-of-the-night sheet changes. The endless cycle of washing, wiping, reassuring, apologising (often on their behalf).

And through it all, you are expected to remain calm, kind, respectful, and endlessly patient.

Which you are.

Until you aren't.

And then you feel guilty for being human.

Let me say this clearly: finding this hard does not make you a bad carer.
It makes you a normal one.

## *THE EMOTIONAL COST NOBODY BUDGETS FOR*

The hardest part of caregiving is not the physical work.

It's the invisible load.

Making decisions no one else wants to make.

Advocating in systems that may not recognise you or your advocacy.

Being "the responsible one" while everyone else lives their lives.

Loving someone who may never say thank you again.

It's loneliness. Even when you're never alone.

It's losing your identity until you're introduced as "the carer" instead of you.

And it's the quiet resentment that creeps in—and then the shame that follows it.

You can love someone deeply and hate how much this has taken from you.

Both things can be true.

## *SO WHY DO WE DO IT?*

After all this, you might ask: Why would anyone do this?

Because love is inconvenient.

Because history matters.

Because sometimes there is no one else.

Because despite everything—the mess, the exhaustion, the heartbreak—there are moments of connection so profound they take your breath away.

- A squeeze of the hand.
- A sudden smile.
- A shared memory that resurfaces like a gift.

And because walking away, for many of us, would hurt more than staying.

## *A WARNING, AND A PROMISE*

So yes—this job is not for the light-hearted.

- It will test you in ways you never imagined.
- It will change you.
- It will age you.

But if you're here—reading this—chances are you've already said yes. Not out loud. Not formally. But with your actions. With your sleepless nights. With your quiet perseverance.
This book is not here to tell you that caregiving is noble or beautiful or easy.

It is here to tell you the truth.

To guide you through the system.

To help you survive it.

And—where possible—to reclaim parts of yourself along the way.

So if you were looking for permission to walk away—take it, if you must.
And if you're staying—then welcome.

Do it if you dare to love someone that much.

# Chapter 2

## *WHEN CARING IS THE JOB*

### *(AND STILL NOT AN EASY ONE)*

Some people fall into caring because love leaves them no other choice.

Others choose it.

- They apply for the job.
- They train.
- They wear uniforms.
- They clock on and off.

And they are often quietly judged by family carers who think, "Well, at least you get paid."

Let's get this out of the way early:

- Being paid does not make caring easy.
- It does not make it light work.
- And it certainly does not make it emotionally neutral.

Choosing aged care as a career is not the "easy option." It is a decision that comes with its own weight, its own heartbreaks, and its own kind of exhaustion.

And without these workers, the entire system would collapse overnight.

## *WHY PEOPLE CHOOSE AGED CARE*

## *(DESPITE EVERYTHING)*

Very few people choose aged care for the money. If they did, they wouldn't stay.

They choose it because:

- They like people
- They believe older lives matter
- They want work with meaning
- They've cared for someone before and felt called to continue
- They have patience, empathy, and a strong stomach—emotionally and physically

Many aged care workers say the same thing in different words:

**"I wanted to make a difference."**

**And they do. Every single day.**

## *THE REALITY BEHIND THE UNIFORM*

On the surface, paid carers have boundaries that family carers don't.
- They go home.
- They have rosters.
- They have employment contracts.

But the work they do within those hours is intense.
They walk into strangers' homes. They step into deeply personal spaces.
They assist with bathing, toileting, dressing, feeding, lifting, and medications—often under time pressure. They meet people on some of the hardest days of their lives. And then they move on to the next client.

## *TIME: THE CONSTANT ENEMY*

One of the biggest challenges for paid carers is time—or the lack of it.
Care plans are written with good intentions, but real life doesn't fit neatly into 30-minute blocks.

You can't rush:

- Dementia confusion
- Anxiety
- Grief
- Pain
- Fear

Yet carers are often expected to:

- Shower someone
- Prepare a meal
- Do basic housework
- Provide companionship
- Document everything

All before the clock runs out.

No matter how kind or skilled you are, time pressure changes the experience of care—for everyone involved.

# *EMOTIONAL LABOUR IS NOT IN THE JOB DESCRIPTION*

## *(BUT IT'S ALWAYS THERE)*

Paid carers are not just performing tasks.

They are:
- Listening to life stories
- Absorbing loneliness
- Witnessing decline
- Comforting people who know they are nearing the end
- Supporting families who are overwhelmed or grieving

They form bonds—because they're human.

And then clients move into residential care. Or pass away.

There is rarely space to grieve. The schedule moves on.
This quiet accumulation of loss is one of the least acknowledged parts of the job.

# DEMENTIA DOES NOT CARE IF YOU'RE PAID

Dementia doesn't soften just because the carer is "professional."

Paid carers are yelled at.

Accused.

Sometimes hit.

Often mistrusted.

They walk into situations where logic no longer applies and compassion must carry the load.

They remain calm when someone is frightened or angry or confused.

They learn not to take it personally—while still caring deeply.

That is not easy work.

## INCONTINENCE, INTIMACY AND DIGNITY

Like family carers, paid carers manage incontinence daily.

What's different is that they do it:
- Repeatedly
- With different people
- In unfamiliar environments

While trying to preserve dignity on both sides

They must be professional and compassionate at the same time.

And they do this knowing that many people feel embarrassed, ashamed, or distressed needing help from a stranger.

Handling that gently takes skill—and heart.

## THE PAY REALITY

Let's be honest. Hourly rates in aged care rarely reflect the responsibility, complexity, and emotional load of the work.

Yes, carers are paid. But they are often:

- Casual or part-time
- Working split shifts
- Juggling multiple employers
- Physically exhausted
- Emotionally drained

Many still struggle financially. This is not "easy money." It is earned—minute by minute.

## WHERE PAID CARERS AND FAMILY CARERS CLASH

There can be tension. Family carers are overwhelmed. Paid carers are stretched thin.

Families sometimes feel:
- Care isn't personal enough
- Workers don't have time
- The system isn't delivering what was promised

Paid carers sometimes feel:
- Micromanaged
- Distrusted
- Emotionally squeezed between policy and reality

And the truth is—both sides are usually right.

The problem is rarely the person doing the caring.

It's the system surrounding them.


## THE GOOD DAYS
## (YES, THEY EXIST)

Despite everything, there are moments that keep people in this work.

A smile.
A thank you.
A familiar face lighting up.
A small win—like a shower completed calmly, or a meal eaten with enjoyment.

These moments matter. They remind carers why they chose this path.

## *BURNOUT IS REAL — AND COMMON*

Aged care workers experience burnout at alarming rates.

- Physical strain.
- Emotional fatigue.
- Compassion exhaustion.

Many leave the sector not because they don't care—but because they care too much, with too little support.

When carers leave, clients lose continuity. Families lose trust. The system strains further. Everyone feels it.


## *WHY RESPECT MATTERS (ON ALL SIDES)*

Family carers and paid carers are not opponents. They are allies—whether they realise it or not.

Both are navigating:
- Decline
- Loss
- Systems that don't flex easily
- Emotional landmines

When respect flows both ways, care improves. When it doesn't, everyone suffers.

## *WHAT THE SYSTEM FORGETS*

The system often forgets that paid carers are people.

- Not just roster numbers.
- Not just task-completers.
- Not just service deliverers.

They bring their own lives, worries, families, and grief into this work. And they still show up.


## *WHY THIS CHAPTER BELONGS IN THIS BOOK*

Because aged care is not just about policies and payments. It's about people caring for people—whether they're related or not.

Understanding the reality of paid carers helps family carers:
- Set realistic expectations
- Build better relationships
- Direct frustration where it belongs (upward, not sideways)

And it helps paid carers feel recognised in a world that often overlooks them.

## THE BOTTOM LINE

Choosing caring as a career doesn't make it easy. It makes it intentional. It comes with pride, purpose, frustration, heartbreak, and moments of deep connection.

Like all caring—it asks more than it gives. And yet, every day, thousands of people choose it anyway.

### THAT DESERVES ACKNOWLEDGMENT!

# Chapter 3

## *HOW THE SYSTEM REALLY WORKS*

### *(AND WHY IT FEELS LIKE IT DOESN'T)*

If caring for someone you love feels hard, wait until you meet the system designed to "help" you.

On paper, Australia's aged care system looks impressive. Structured. Regulated. Full of pathways, portals, and well-meaning acronyms. There are flow charts and phone numbers and government websites promising choice, support, and navigation.

In real life, it feels like being dropped into a maze while blindfolded, exhausted, and already grieving.

No one sits you down at the beginning and explains how this works. There's no orientation session. No starter pack. No calm professional saying, "Here's what's going to happen, and here's how we'll help you through it."

Instead, you learn the system the same way you learn everything else as a carer: the hard way.

### *THE FIRST LIE: "HELP IS AVAILABLE"*

Help is available—but not immediately, not easily, and not without persistence.
The system assumes you:
- Have time
- Have energy
- Have internet access
- Can sit on hold for long periods
- Can absorb complex information while emotionally overwhelmed

Carers rarely tick all those boxes. You usually enter the system at crisis point. A hospital discharge. A fall. A diagnosis. A moment when it becomes painfully clear that life has changed—and you're expected to catch up quickly. That's when someone casually says, "Have you contacted My Aged Care?" As if that's a single phone call, neatly resolved.

## *MY AGED CARE: THE FRONT DOOR*
## *(WITH A VERY LONG HALLWAY)*

My Aged Care is the official entry point to government-funded aged care. It's the front door.

But it's not a warm, welcoming one.

It's a door that opens into a long corridor of assessments, waiting lists, eligibility criteria, and referrals—many of which don't move at the pace of real life.

You call. You explain your situation. You repeat yourself. You answer questions that feel oddly disconnected from reality.

Can they shower independently?
Can they prepare meals?
Do they feel safe at home?

You answer honestly, because you're exhausted and hopeful. Then you wait.

And this is where carers begin to realise a fundamental truth:

The system moves slowly. Illness does not.

## *ASSESSMENTS*

### *NECESSARY, BUT NEVER NEUTRAL*

Assessments are essential. They determine eligibility, funding, and access to services. Without them, nothing happens. But assessments are not the same as understanding.

A stranger—usually kind, sometimes rushed—comes into your home or hospital room and tries to capture a complex human life in a checklist. They see a snapshot. You live the full picture.

They may not see the nights without sleep. The emotional volatility. The sheer effort it takes to keep everything running.

And because many carers minimise—because that's what carers do—needs are often underplayed. We say, "We're managing," when what we mean is, "We're barely holding this together." And the system believes what it hears.

### *WAITING LISTS: THE QUIET BREAKING POINT*

This is where the system truly starts to feel like it's failing you. You can be approved for support—and still wait months, sometimes years, to receive it. Home Care Packages are the biggest example. You're assessed. You're approved. You're told help is coming. And then you wait.

Meanwhile, your caring responsibilities increase. Your health declines. Your world shrinks. The system assumes you'll somehow bridge the gap. Most carers do—at great personal cost.

## *CHOICE, BUT ONLY IF YOU'RE RESILIENT ENOUGH TO CHASE IT*

We're told the system offers choice and control. And it does—if you have the capacity to research, compare providers, read fine print, negotiate fees, and advocate relentlessly.

But carers are often doing this at midnight, after everyone else is asleep.

You become:
- A researcher
- A contract reader
- A negotiator
- A scheduler
- A complaint writer

All while performing intimate, emotionally taxing care. The system doesn't assign you a guide. It assumes you'll become one.

## *THE LANGUAGE BARRIER NOBODY TALKS ABOUT*

The aged care system speaks a language of policy. Carers speak the language of love and crisis.

Words like consumer, service delivery, co-contribution, and care plan don't reflect the lived reality of holding someone while they cry because they don't recognise their own home.

The system isn't cruel—but it is clinical.

And when you're operating from the heart, that disconnect hurts.

## WHY IT FEELS LIKE YOU'RE ALWAYS DOING SOMETHING WRONG

One of the most corrosive aspects of the system is how often carers feel they've failed—when they haven't.

Miss a form?
Didn't know you had to reapply?
Didn't chase a referral fast enough?

Suddenly services stop, payments are delayed, or help never arrives.

And because the system doesn't see the full weight you're carrying, the burden falls back on you.

Again.


## THE UNSPOKEN ASSUMPTION: THAT YOU'LL JUST KEEP GOING

At its core, the system relies heavily on unpaid carers. It works because you do.

Every gap is filled by love. Every delay absorbed by sacrifice.

And while there is gratitude in theory, in practice carers often feel invisible—until something goes wrong.

The system does not collapse because carers hold it up. But carers often collapse quietly, off to the side.

## *WHY THIS ISN'T YOUR FAULT*

If the system feels confusing, slow and exhausting, it's not because you're doing it wrong. It's because it wasn't designed around the lived reality of caregiving.

It was designed in departments. Written in legislation. Implemented through layers of administration.

You're not failing the system. The system is struggling to keep up with you.

## *LEARNING TO WORK THE SYSTEM*
## *(WITHOUT LOSING YOURSELF)*

Over time, carers develop survival skills:
- Document everything
- Ask for names
- Follow up
- Advocate firmly
- Accept help when it finally arrives

This book will help you do that—with clarity, not guilt.

But hear this now, before we go any further:
You are not weak for finding this hard.
You are not ungrateful for wanting more support.
And you are not alone in feeling like this shouldn't be so difficult.

## *WHAT THIS CHAPTER WANTS YOU TO KNOW*

The aged care system is not your enemy—but it is not your saviour either.

It can help. It can support. But it requires persistence, patience, and knowledge you were never formally given.

That's why this handbook exists.

Not to tell you to "be grateful." But to help you navigate, protect yourself, and survive the long haul. Because caring is already hard enough.

The system should not be the hardest part.

## *BEFORE YOU DO ANYTHING ELSE*

Before we go any further—before the paperwork, the assessments, the packages, the laws, and the endless acronyms—we need to stop.

Not forever.
Not dramatically.
Just long enough to ask a question that the system almost never asks:

How are you doing?

Not the polite version.
Not the "I'm fine" you give out of habit.
The real answer.

Because if the carer collapses, everything collapses.

And yet, carers are consistently treated as an unlimited resource—emotionally, physically, and psychologically.

This chapter exists to say what no form ever does:

You matter in this equation.

## *THE CARER AS INFRASTRUCTURE*
## *(WHETHER YOU LIKE IT OR NOT)*

Here's an uncomfortable truth: The aged care system is built on carers.

Unpaid carers.
Underpaid carers.
Exhausted carers.

You are not just part of the picture—you are the scaffolding holding everything up.

Every gap in service delivery?
You fill it.

Every delay in funding?
You absorb it.

Every assumption that "someone will manage"?
That someone is you.

But unlike buildings, carers are not designed to carry infinite load without cracking.

## *WHY BURNOUT ISN'T A PERSONAL FAILURE*

Carer burnout is often spoken about in hushed tones, as though it's something shameful.

It isn't.

Burnout is not weakness.
It is not poor coping.
It is not a failure of love.

Burnout is what happens when responsibility exceeds support for too long.

And carers are uniquely vulnerable because:
- The work is relentless
- The emotional stakes are high
- The role is poorly defined
- There is no natural "off switch"

You cannot clock out of loving someone who needs you.


## *THE EARLY WARNING SIGNS WE IGNORE*

Burnout doesn't usually arrive with flashing lights. It creeps in quietly. You might notice:
- You're constantly tired, even after sleeping
- You feel irritable or numb
- You cry unexpectedly—or not at all
- You dread mornings
- You fantasise about escape and then feel guilty for it
- Your own health appointments keep getting postponed
- You tell yourself, "I'll deal with this later"—and later never comes

Many carers don't recognise burnout because they're still functioning. Functioning is not thriving.

## THE MYTH OF "I CAN HANDLE IT"

Carers are problem-solvers by necessity.

When something needs doing, you do it.
When something breaks, you fix it.
When help doesn't arrive, you step in.

Over time, this creates a dangerous narrative:

"If I don't do it, no one will."

Sometimes that's true. But believing it absolutely is how carers disappear.


## WHY SELF-CARE IS THE WRONG WORD
## (BUT THE RIGHT IDEA)

Let's be honest—self-care has a branding problem.

It's been reduced to bubble baths, candles, and yoga poses that feel wildly out of reach when you're changing sheets at 2am.

What carers need is not indulgence. They need maintenance.

Think of it this way:
You are essential equipment. If a piece of equipment is critical to operations, you don't wait until it breaks to look after it.

You maintain it. You service it. You protect it. Caring for yourself is not selfish. It is care continuity planning.

## THE GUILT TRAP

Carer guilt is powerful—and deeply unfair.

Guilt tells you:
- You're not doing enough
- You should be more patient
- You shouldn't complain
- Others have it worse
- Wanting a break makes you ungrateful

Guilt thrives in silence.

And the system benefits from it—because guilty carers don't ask for more.

Let's be clear:

Feeling overwhelmed does not mean you love less.
Wanting rest does not mean you're abandoning anyone.
Needing help does not mean you've failed.

## THE COST OF IGNORING YOURSELF

When carers don't protect themselves, the consequences ripple outward.

- Health deteriorates
- Depression and anxiety increase
- Relationships suffer
- Financial stress deepens
- Decisions get harder
- Resentment builds

Eventually, the care situation reaches crisis point—often suddenly, often traumatically
Preventing crisis is not a luxury. It is a strategy.

## *WHAT PROTECTING THE CARER*
## *ACTUALLY LOOKS LIKE*

Protecting yourself doesn't mean dramatic life overhauls. It means small, intentional acts of preservation.

It might look like:
- Attending your own medical appointments
- Saying no to one extra task
- Asking for respite before you're desperate
- Documenting instead of remembering everything
- Letting a service do a job imperfectly rather than doing it yourself perfectly
- Naming when something is too much

## *PROTECTION IS PRACTICAL.*
## *BOUNDARIES ARE NOT CRUEL*

Carers are often afraid of boundaries because they feel like abandonment. They aren't. Boundaries are the framework that makes care sustainable.

A boundary might be:
- "I can't do nights anymore."
- "I need help with showering tasks."
- "I can't manage appointments alone."
- "I need a break, even if nothing has changed."

Boundaries don't mean you care less. They mean you intend to last longer.

## *THE ROLE NO ONE PREPARED YOU FOR*

Most carers didn't choose this role. And even those who did weren't trained for the emotional complexity of it.

You are:
- Advocate
- Coordinator
- Witness
- Buffer
- Translator between systems and humans
- Holder of history
- Keeper of dignity

That is a lot for one person.

Acknowledging that is not weakness.

It is honesty.


## *REST IS NOT EARNED*

Carers often believe rest must be justified.

- Once this is sorted.
- Once they're stable.
- Once the paperwork is done.

But care rarely reaches a neat stopping point. If you wait for permission to rest, you may never get it.

Rest is not a reward. It is a requirement.

## ASKING FOR HELP BEFORE YOU'RE DESPERATE

One of the hardest lessons carers learn is this:

If you wait until you're drowning, help arrives too late—or not at all.

The system responds better to planning than crisis.

Protecting yourself early:
- Strengthens assessments
- Improves outcomes
- Preserves relationships
- Keeps you healthier

You are allowed to say:
"I'm not coping,"
even if you're still functioning.

## WHAT THIS CHAPTER IS GIVING YOU
## PERMISSION TO DO

This chapter gives you permission to:
- Take yourself seriously
- Acknowledge the toll
- Stop minimising your needs
- Seek support early
- Care for yourself without apology

Because everything that follows in this book—every form, every package, every decision—depends on you being able to keep going. And not just keep going. Keep going without losing yourself.

## *BEFORE WE MOVE ON*

Before the next chapter pulls you back into the mechanics of the system, pause.

Take a breath.

Notice your body.
Notice your exhaustion.
Notice how long it's been since anyone asked how you were coping.

You don't need to fix everything today. But you do need to stay in the picture.

## *LOOKING AHEAD*

The next chapters will help you:
- Navigate assessments more effectively
- Use the system without being crushed by it
- Advocate clearly and firmly
- Make informed decisions without constant guilt
- But none of that matters if you disappear along the way.

**So we start here.**

**With you.**

# Chapter 4

## *ASSESSMENTS WITHOUT TEARS*

### *(OR AT LEAST FEWER OF THEM)*

If assessments came with warning labels, they'd read something like this:

May cause emotional exhaustion, guilt, frustration and the urge to scream into the nearest pillow.

Assessments are unavoidable. They are the gateway to support. And under the new aged care legislation, they are meant to be fairer, more humane, and more respectful of both the older person and the carer.

That's the intention.

This chapter exists to help you navigate the reality—without breaking down in the process.

## *WHAT THE NEW AGED CARE LAWS SAY*
## *(AND WHY THAT MATTERS TO YOU)*

Australia's new aged care legislation marks a significant shift. For the first time, the system is explicitly rights-based.

Older people are recognised as rights holders—not passive recipients of services. And crucially, carers are formally acknowledged as part of the care relationship, not just background helpers. Under the new Act and reforms:
- Wellbeing is central, not optional
- Dignity of risk is recognised
- Supported decision-making replaces default substitute decision-making
- Carers' insights are meant to be considered
- Assessments are supposed to be person-centred, not box-ticking exercises

On paper, this is a major improvement.

In practice, it still depends heavily on:
- The assessor
- The time allocated
- How clearly needs are expressed
- How well carers advocate

Which brings us to the emotional reality.

## *WHY ASSESSMENTS FEEL SO AWFUL*

## *(EVEN WHEN THEY'RE DONE "WELL")*

Assessments require you to do something deeply uncomfortable: Expose the cracks in someone you love. You are asked to describe:
- What they can no longer do
- Where they are unsafe
- How much they rely on you
- What is going wrong behind closed doors

This can feel:
- Disloyal
- Cruel
- Like you're taking away their independence

And when dementia is involved, it can feel downright brutal. The new legislation recognises psychological safety and dignity, but the process still asks carers to narrate decline. There's no way to make that painless.

# SUPPORTED DECISION-MAKING

## WHAT IT MEANS FOR ASSESSMENTS

One of the most important changes under the new laws is the emphasis on supported decision-making. This means:
- Older people are presumed capable of making decisions
- Support should be provided to help them understand and express choices
- Decisions should reflect their values, not just clinical risk

For carers, this can feel like a double-edged sword.

On one hand:
- It protects autonomy
- It reduces paternalism
- It respects identity

On the other:
- It can place carers in a difficult position when safety is already compromised
- It can feel like reality is being politely ignored

Your role in assessments is not to override the person—but to contextualise their answers. You are allowed to say:
"With support, this is possible—but without it, it isn't." That distinction matters.

# THE CARER'S VOICE

## RECOGNISED IN LAW, OFTEN OVERLOOKED IN PRACTICE

The new Act explicitly acknowledges carers as:
- Contributors to care
- Holders of critical information
- People whose wellbeing impacts care outcomes

That is huge. But recognition does not automatically translate into protection.

Assessors may still:
- Focus primarily on the older person
- Underestimate the carer's workload
- Assume support will continue indefinitely

You may need to assert your presence respectfully but firmly.
- You are not "interfering."
- You are providing essential context.

## PREPARING FOR AN ASSESSMENT

## THE KINDEST THING YOU CAN DO

Preparation is not manipulation. It is survival. Before an assessment:
- Write notes (do not rely on memory)
- Track difficult days—not just good ones
- List what you are doing to keep things afloat
- Identify what would break first if you stepped back

Assessments tend to focus on tasks. You need to highlight effort. Instead of: "Yes, they shower." Try: "They shower because I prompt, supervise, assist, and manage safety."

This aligns with the new well being-focused framework, which looks at sustainability—not just capacity.

## WHAT NOT TO MINIMISE

## (EVEN IF IT FEELS UNKIND)

Carers instinctively soften the truth. We say:
- "It's not that bad."
- "We're managing."
- "I don't want to make a fuss."

The system hears:
No urgency. No risk. No need.

Under the new legislation, assessors are meant to consider carer strain and sustainability. But they can't assess what you don't disclose. You are not betraying anyone by being honest. You are planning for safety.

## WHEN THE PERSON YOU CARE FOR

## DISAGREES WITH YOU

This is one of the most distressing parts of assessments.
The person may say:
- "I don't need help."
- "I do everything myself."
- "They're exaggerating."

Especially with cognitive decline, this creates tension—and sometimes anger.

The new Act encourages supported communication, but it does not require carers to pretend everything is fine.

You can calmly state: "That's their experience. Mine is different." Both can be true.

## WHY ASSESSMENTS STILL FEEL RUSHED

Despite legislative reform, assessments are still constrained by:
- Workforce shortages
- Time limits
- Administrative pressure

This is not a reflection of your worth. It is a structural issue. If you feel unheard:
- Ask for clarification
- Request notes be recorded
- Follow up in writing
- 

Documentation matters more than emotion in the system—even when emotion is driving the need.

## AFTER THE ASSESSMENT

## THE EMOTIONAL CRASH

Many carers report a strange emotional drop after assessments. You hold it together. You perform competence. You advocate. Then it's over—and you feel empty, guilty, or shattered. This is normal. You have just:
- Publicly acknowledged loss
- Asked for help
- Exposed vulnerability

Be gentle with yourself.

The new legislation speaks of trauma-informed care. That includes you—even if the system forgets that sometimes.

## *APPROVAL IS NOT SUPPORT*
## *(BUT IT IS LEVERAGE)*

Even under the reformed system, approval does not equal immediate help. But it does give you:
- Standing
- Language
- Legitimacy

Once approved, you can:
- Advocate with evidence
- Escalate with clarity

Say, "This has already been assessed as necessary." The new Act strengthens your position here. Use it.

## *REASSESSMENTS ARE NOT FAILURES*

Under the new framework, reassessment is expected when:
- Needs change
- Care becomes unsustainable
- Carer wellbeing declines

Requesting reassessment does not mean the system failed. It means life changed. And life always does.

## WHAT THIS CHAPTER WANTS YOU TO REMEMBER

Assessments are emotionally taxing because they ask you to name loss.

The new aged care laws recognise dignity, wellbeing, and carer involvement.

Your voice is legitimate—even when it feels uncomfortable.

Preparation is not deceit; it is clarity.

Tears are allowed—but so is strength.

The system is slowly changing.

Your need is immediate.

Both truths coexist.

## LOOKING AHEAD

The next chapter will tackle:
- Payments
- Fees
- Means testing

And why "support" still often costs carers more than it gives.

But for now, know this:

You are not weak for finding assessments hard.

You are doing one of the hardest things there is—telling the truth about care.

And that truth is the first step toward support that actually works.

# Chapter 5

## *WHEN THE CARER BECOMES INVISIBLE*

### *A CASE STUDY*

This is not an unusual story. It is not an extreme case. It is not a one-off.

It is a quiet example of what happens when systems focus on process over people — and when the carer, despite being central to the care arrangement, effectively disappears from view.

### *THE SITUATION*

An older woman in her early seventies was living with multiple serious health conditions, including end-stage chronic renal failure. Following a hospital admission for pneumonia, she experienced a noticeable cognitive decline. Over time, symptoms consistent with dementia became increasingly apparent.

At home, she relied heavily on one person — her primary carer — for day-to-day support, safety, and coordination of care. This person managed appointments, medication oversight, daily living tasks, and emotional support. Without this involvement, the care arrangement would not have been sustainable.

Anticipating future decline, the older woman had previously signed an Enduring Power of Attorney (EPOA), appointing her trusted carer as her substitute decision-maker if capacity was lost. She had also completed an Aged Care Directive outlining her wishes regarding medical treatment, including a clear preference for no antibiotics, although the directive had not yet been formally signed. At this point, the arrangement was fragile but functioning.

## *THE HOSPITAL ADMISSION*

## *A MISSED OPPORTUNITY*

The older woman was admitted to hospital with double pneumonia and remained there for approximately ten days.

During this admission:
- The primary carer was not consulted regarding treatment decisions There was no discussion about the home environment she would be discharged into
- No one contacted the carer to assess whether discharge would be safe or sustainable

Despite the presence of an Aged Care Directive expressing clear treatment preferences (albeit unsigned at this stage), no one sought clarification from the person holding the EPOA or discussed whether substitute decision-making should be activated.

In hindsight, this was a critical moment.

At this point:
- Cognitive impairment was evident
- Acute illness was compounding chronic conditions
- Decision-making capacity was likely compromised

Yet no one asked whether the EPOA should be invoked. No one asked who would manage care on discharge. The carer remained invisible.

## RETURN HOME & DECLINE

After discharge, the older woman returned home. Her cognitive state had worsened. Confusion increased. Behaviour became unpredictable. The primary carer absorbed the escalating demands and attempted to stabilise the situation without formal support.

She phoned the hospital twice to ask what the discharge plan was. She was told that the patient is no longer in our care, and your questions should be referred to her GP.

The system had already assumed: "Someone is managing." That assumption was incorrect — but unchallenged.


## THE REASSESSMENT

A reassessment was later triggered through the aged care system to review the woman's care needs. The reassessment was conducted via phone.

The primary carer — the person providing daily support and holding critical information about safety, behaviour, and functional decline — was not included.

- No in-person visit occurred.
- No direct observation of the living environment took place.
- No carer interview was conducted.

As a result, the reassessment relied largely on self-report.

## WHAT WAS MISSED

Without carer input, several critical factors were not adequately captured:

The extent of cognitive impairment
- Emerging delusional beliefs
- Behavioural changes affecting safety
- The increasing emotional and physical strain on the care arrangement
- The degree to which independence was being propped up by constant supervision

On paper, the situation appeared more stable than it actually was.

In reality, it was deteriorating rapidly.

## ESCALATION AND BREAKDOWN

Following the reassessment, the situation escalated sharply.

The older woman began expressing fixed beliefs that her carer was attempting to harm her. These beliefs were communicated to service providers and medical professionals. The allegations were serious and emotionally charged, but they arose in the context of documented cognitive decline.

At this point, the care arrangement crossed from "difficult" into unsafe.

The primary carer, faced with delusional accusations and no additional supports, made the decision to leave the care environment in order to protect personal safety.

This decision was not abandonment. It was a safety response.

## INVOKING THE EPOA

Around this time, the Enduring Power of Attorney was formally invoked.

A written medical opinion from the woman's long-term GP stated that she lacked decision-making capacity regarding health and care decisions due to both acute and chronic medical conditions, including dementia.

Under the law, this should have triggered:
- recognition of the substitute decision-maker
- safeguarding processes
- structured reassessment of capacity and risk

Instead, something else occurred.

## WHEN LEGAL AUTHORITY IS QUIETLY SET ASIDE

Despite the medical confirmation of incapacity, the EPOA was not recognised in practice.

Service providers and clinicians continued to rely on statements made by the older woman during a period of compromised cognition. The substitute decision-maker was excluded from further decision-making and consultation.

- No formal capacity reassessment occurred.
- No safeguarding review was initiated.
- No independent investigation into the allegations was undertaken.

The EPOA was not formally revoked — it was simply ignored.

## THE OUTCOME

The older woman remained living alone.

Despite clear evidence that she required continuous supervision and support, no immediate alternative care arrangement was put in place. The collapse of the informal care arrangement was treated as a personal issue, rather than a predictable system failure.

What had been holding the situation together — the invisible labour of the carer — was gone.

And the system struggled to respond.

## WHAT THIS CASE REVEALS

This case highlights several systemic issues that carers encounter repeatedly:

- Carer invisibility often begins in hospital settings
- Failure to include carers during admission and discharge planning sets the stage for later breakdown.
- Advance care planning is ineffective if carers are excluded
- Directives and EPOAs cannot guide care if the people holding them are not consulted.
- Phone-based assessments are inadequate for complex cognitive cases - They rely too heavily on self-report and cannot capture behavioural risk or delusional thinking.
- Legal safeguards are only effective if they are honoured
- An EPOA is meaningless if it can be sidelined without due process.
- Carer safety is still poorly embedded in practice
- Abuse and delusional accusations are often minimised until a crisis occurs.

## THE INVISIBLE CARER PROBLEM

Throughout this case, the carer appears only at the margins:
- not present in hospital decision-making
- not consulted in discharge planning
- not included in assessments
- not protected when risk escalated

Yet the system depended on this person entirely.

This is the paradox of caring:
- carers are essential — until they are inconvenient.

When carers are invisible, systems make poor decisions.


## WHY THIS MATTERS FOR OTHER CARERS

This case is not included to alarm. It is included to prepare.

Carers need to know:
- exclusion during hospital admissions is a warning sign
- discharge without consultation is a risk factor
- advance care documents are only as strong as their recognition
- EPOAs must be actively engaged, not assumed
- safety trumps obligation

Most importantly, carers need permission to step away when safety is lost.

## THE LESSON

When carers are invisible, risk increases.

Not just for carers — but for the people they are trying to protect.

This chapter is not about blame. It is about recognising that care does not exist in isolation. It is relational, contextual and fragile. Remove one part of that structure without replacing it, and everything else is at risk.

## LOOKING AHEAD

In the next chapter, we move from story to strategy:
- how to make yourself visible early
- how to assert your role in hospital settings
- how to activate safeguards before crisis
- and how to step back safely when systems fail

Because the goal is not to scare carers. It is to ensure they are never erased.

# MAPPING THE CASE TO THE NEW AGED CARE ACT
## WHERE THE SYSTEM FAILED ITS OWN OBLIGATIONS

Australia's new Aged Care Act was designed to prevent exactly the kind of situation described in this case study. It introduces a rights-based framework that centres dignity, safety, wellbeing and recognition of carers as integral to care arrangements.

When this case is viewed through that lens, the gaps become clear.

**1. Obligation: Person-Centred and Wellbeing-Focused Care - What the Act requires:**
The new Aged Care Act places wellbeing at the centre of all decision-making. Care planning and assessment must consider not only physical health, but psychological safety, cognitive capacity, and the sustainability of care arrangements.

**What happened in this case:**
- Cognitive decline following hospitalisation was not adequately assessed in context
- Behavioural changes and delusional beliefs were not factored into care planning
- The emotional and psychological safety of both the older person and the carer were overlooked

**Why this matters:**
Wellbeing cannot be assessed in isolation. When care relies on one person, that relationship must be examined. Ignoring it undermines the Act's core intent.

**2. Obligation: Recognition of Carers as Key Participants - What the Act requires:**
Carers are explicitly recognised as key contributors to care. Their insights must be considered in assessments, reassessments, and care planning, particularly where care sustainability and safety are concerned.

**What happened in this case:**
- The primary carer was excluded from hospital discussions
- The carer was not consulted during discharge planning
- The carer was not included in the ACAT reassessment
- Decisions were made as if care existed independently of the carer
- 
-

**Why this matters:**
The system relied on the carer's labour while simultaneously excluding their voice. This directly contradicts the Act's requirement to recognise carers as central, not peripheral.

### 3. Obligation: Safe and Appropriate Discharge Planning - What the Act requires:
Under the new framework, transitions between care settings — particularly hospital discharge — must include planning for safety, continuity of care, and the capacity of informal supports. This includes:
- confirming the home environment is safe
- identifying who will provide care
- assessing whether informal care is sustainable

**What happened in this case:**
- No consultation occurred during a ten-day hospital admission
- No check was made regarding the safety or sustainability of discharge
- No assessment was undertaken of the carer's capacity to continue
- The assumption that "someone will manage" went unchallenged

**Why this matters:**
Unsafe discharge planning is a known trigger for care breakdown. The Act seeks to prevent this by embedding shared responsibility. That responsibility was not exercised here.

### 4. Obligation: Supported Decision-Making (With Safeguards) - What the Act requires:
Supported decision-making replaces automatic substitute decision-making, but only where capacity exists. Where capacity is impaired, safeguards must activate.
Supported decision-making does not mean:
- accepting all statements at face value
- ignoring evidence of cognitive impairment
- side-lining legally appointed decision-makers

**What happened in this case:**
- Statements made during delusional episodes were relied upon
- Allegations arising from cognitive impairment were not independently reviewed
- Capacity was not reassessed when behaviour escalated

**Why this matters:**
The Act balances autonomy with protection. In this case, autonomy was privileged without adequate assessment, increasing risk rather than reducing it.

**5. Obligation: Recognition of Enduring Power of Attorney - What the Act requires:**
Where an Enduring Power of Attorney is invoked, the substitute decision-maker must be recognised and consulted unless formally set aside through appropriate legal or safeguarding processes.

**What happened in this case:**
The EPOA was validly invoked with medical confirmation of incapacity. Despite this, the EPOA was disregarded in practice. No formal capacity reassessment or safeguarding investigation occurred. The EPOA was effectively ignored rather than reviewed.

**Why this matters:**
The Act does not allow informal rejection of legal authority. Ignoring an EPOA without due process undermines trust in advance planning and exposes vulnerable people to risk.

**6. Obligation: Safeguarding When Risk Emerges - What the Act requires:**
When care arrangements become unsafe — including situations involving abuse, delusional beliefs, or breakdown of informal care — safeguarding processes must be triggered.

**What happened in this case:**
- Delusional accusations against the carer were treated as credible without investigation
- No safeguarding review occurred
- The carer was left unprotected
- The older person was left without adequate care

**Why this matters:**
Safeguarding is not optional. It exists to protect both the person receiving care and those involved in providing it.

## THE CENTRAL FAILURE

## THE CARER WAS TREATED AS OPTIONAL

Across hospital care, discharge planning, reassessment, and safeguarding, the same pattern repeated:
- The carer was essential
- The carer was relied upon
- The carer was not consulted
- The carer was not protected

This is precisely what the new Aged Care Act is meant to change.


## WHY THIS MAPPING MATTERS

This case is not about individual mistakes. It is about what happens when:
- legislation changes faster than practice
- carers are named in policy but ignored on the ground
- systems still operate as if care is infinite and invisible

By mapping lived experience directly to legislative obligations, carers can:
- recognise when the system is failing them
- name those failures clearly
- advocate with confidence rather than apology

## *LOOKING FORWARD*

The intent of the new Aged Care Act is sound. But intent only matters if it is enacted.

The chapters that follow will focus on:
- how carers can insist on inclusion early
- how to reference the Act in real conversations
- how to trigger safeguards before crisis
- and how to step back safely when obligations are not met

Because recognition in law must become recognition in practice.

**And carers should never again be invisible.**

# Chapter 6

## *CARER VISIBILITY CHECKLIST*

### For Hospital Admissions, Discharge Planning & Aged Care Assessments

**Purpose:**
To help carers ensure they are recognised, consulted, and protected — and that care decisions are safe, lawful, and sustainable. You do not need to tick every box. You do not need to be "difficult." You are allowed to ask these questions.

## *AT HOSPITAL ADMISSION*

**Ask early — don't wait for discharge.**
☐ Have I clearly identified myself as the primary carer?
☐ Has my name and contact number been recorded in the medical file?
☐ Have staff asked who provides day-to-day care at home?
☐ Have they asked whether the home environment is safe and sustainable?

**If there is cognitive impairment:**
☐ Has anyone assessed or documented decision-making capacity?
☐ Has delirium, dementia, or confusion been noted?
☐ Have changes in behaviour been communicated to me?

**If there is an EPOA or Advance Care Directive:**
☐ Have I informed staff that an EPOA exists?
☐ Have I provided a copy (or told them where to obtain it)?
☐ Has anyone asked whether the EPOA should be invoked?
☐ Has the Advance/Aged Care Directive been reviewed or discussed?
Red flag: If no one asks who will manage care after discharge, the system is already assuming the carer will cope.

## *DURING HOSPITAL STAY*

☐ Am I being included in discussions about treatment and care planning?

□ Have staff checked in with me about how the person is managing at home?
□ Have changes in cognition or behaviour been escalated, not minimised?

**If the person makes allegations or shows paranoia/delusions:**

□ Has this been documented as a possible cognitive/behavioural issue?
□ Has capacity been reassessed or flagged for review?
□ Has safeguarding been discussed?

You can say:
"This behaviour is new and out of character. I'm concerned about capacity and safety."

## *DISCHARGE PLANNING (CRITICAL SECTION)*

□ Has anyone asked whether discharge home is safe?
□ Has anyone confirmed who will provide care?
□ Has the sustainability of informal care been assessed?
□ Have community supports been organised before discharge?

If you are the carer:

□ Have I been asked if I can realistically continue caring?
□ Have I been offered respite, support, or follow-up?
□ Has my wellbeing been considered at all?

You are allowed to say: "I cannot safely manage this level of care without support."

# AGED CARE ASSESSMENTS

## (RAS / ACAT / ACAS)

☐ Have I been included in the assessment?
☐ Has the assessment been conducted in person where cognition is impaired?
☐ Has reliance on the carer been clearly documented?
Be careful not to minimise:

☐ Have I explained what I do, not just what the person "can" do?
☐ Have I described difficult days, not just good ones?
☐ Have I been honest about exhaustion, stress, or safety concerns?

Instead of: "They can shower."
Say: "They shower because I supervise and assist to prevent falls."

## CAPACITY, BEHAVIOUR & SAFETY

☐ Has capacity been formally assessed or reviewed?
☐ Have delusions, paranoia, or aggression been documented appropriately?
☐ Has anyone asked whether the care arrangement is still safe?

If abuse occurs (verbal, emotional, physical):
☐ Have I named it as a safety issue?
☐ Have I asked what safeguarding steps will be taken?
☐ Have I been told I am allowed to step back if unsafe?

**Important:**
**Abuse is never an expected part of caring.**

## ENDURING POWER OF ATTORNEY (EPOA)

☐ Is the EPOA on file and recognised?
☐ If invoked, am I being consulted as the substitute decision-maker?
☐ If not consulted, has anyone explained why?
☐ Has any rejection of the EPOA followed proper legal or safeguarding processes?

Red flag:
An EPOA cannot be ignored informally. It must be recognised or formally reviewed.


## IF YOU ARE BEING IGNORED

If you feel invisible, ask calmly:

☐ "Can you please record my concerns in the notes?"
☐ "Who is responsible for ensuring carer wellbeing is considered?"
☐ "What is the escalation pathway if care becomes unsafe?"
☐ "Can we pause this decision until the carer is included?"

If needed, request:
☐ A reassessment
☐ A safeguarding review
☐ A different assessor
☐ Written confirmation of decisions

## PERMISSION (THIS MATTERS)

☐ I am allowed to speak up
☐ I am allowed to say I'm not coping
☐ I am allowed to insist on inclusion
☐ I am allowed to leave if it becomes unsafe

The system may move slowly. Your safety does not have to.

## FINAL REMINDER FOR CARERS

If you are invisible:
- assessments are incomplete
- decisions are unsafe
- and everyone is at risk

The new Aged Care Act recognises carers as essential.

This checklist helps make that recognition real.

# Chapter 7

## *MAKING YOURSELF VISIBLE*

### *(WITHOUT BEING LABELLED "DIFFICULT")*

Most carers don't stay silent because they don't know something is wrong.
They stay silent because they are afraid of what will happen if they speak.

- Afraid of being dismissed.
- Afraid of being labelled "difficult."
- Afraid that services will withdraw.
- Afraid that making noise will make things worse.

The new Aged Care Act was designed to change this dynamic. It explicitly recognises carers, embeds wellbeing and safety, and shifts responsibility back onto systems — not individuals. But legislation alone doesn't change conversations.

This chapter is about how carers speak up in real settings — hospitals, assessments, service meetings — without burning bridges or themselves.

## *WHY CARERS BECOME INVISIBLE*

Carers don't disappear accidentally. They disappear because they are:
- polite
- tired
- grateful for any help
- used to coping

The system often mistakes functioning for capacity. If you show up organised, calm, and capable, the system assumes: "They've got this." Under the new Aged Care Act, this assumption is no longer acceptable.

# WHAT THE NEW AGED CARE ACT ACTUALLY SAYS
## (IN PLAIN ENGLISH)

The Act introduces several principles that matter directly to carers:
- Wellbeing is central, not optional
- Carers are recognised contributors, not bystanders
- Care must be sustainable, not just possible today
- Safeguards must activate when risk emerges
- Decision-making must reflect capacity, not convenience

This means: If the carer collapses, the system has failed. Your role is not to convince people you're struggling — it's to name risk in a way the system is required to hear.

# REFRAMING ADVOCACY
## WHAT IT IS (AND ISN'T)

Let's be clear about what advocacy is not. Advocacy is not:
- complaining
- being rude
- threatening legal action
- demanding perfection

Advocacy is:
- naming safety issues
- clarifying responsibility
- asking for documentation
- insisting on inclusion
- slowing decisions that are unsafe

Under the Act, this is not optional behaviour. It is participation.

## THE CARER'S VOICE

## FROM EMOTION TO AUTHORITY

Carers are often dismissed when they speak emotionally — even when the emotion is justified. The key is not to suppress emotion, but to translate it into system language. Instead of: "I can't cope anymore."

Try: "This care arrangement is no longer sustainable without additional support."
Both are true. Only one activates obligation.


## HOW TO MAKE YOURSELF VISIBLE EARLY

Use these phrases before things escalate.

"I'm the primary carer, and I need to be included in all discussions about care and discharge."

"My ability to continue caring is part of the risk assessment."

"Can you please document that I've raised concerns about sustainability and safety?"

"Who is responsible for ensuring carer wellbeing is considered under the current framework?"

- These are calm.
- They are factual.
- They are very hard to ignore.

## WHY 'DIFFICULT' IS A MYTH
## (AND A CONVENIENT ONE)

The fear of being labelled "difficult" keeps carers quiet. But here's the uncomfortable truth:

Carers who say nothing are easy — until the system collapses.

The Act does not require carers to be agreeable. It requires systems to be accountable.

A carer who asks for documentation, clarity, and safety is not difficult. They are doing exactly what the legislation anticipates.


## WHEN YOU ARE BEING IGNORED

If your concerns are brushed aside:
"I'm not asking for a decision right now. I'm asking for this to be documented."

"If this proceeds without my input, can you explain how carer safety has been considered?"

"What is the escalation pathway if this care arrangement fails?"

Silence is often used to deflect responsibility.

Documentation removes that option.

# MAPPING ADVOCACY TO THE NEW AGED CARE ACT

## OBLIGATION: RECOGNITION OF CARERS

**The Act explicitly recognises carers as contributors to care planning and decision-making.**

What that means in practice:
- You are entitled to be included in assessments
- Your input is relevant evidence
- Excluding you creates an incomplete assessment

What you can say:
"The Act recognises carers as key contributors. I need my input reflected in this assessment."


## OBLIGATION: SUSTAINABLE CARE ARRANGEMENTS

Care is not compliant if it relies on burnout.

What that means:
- "Managing" is not the same as "sustainable"
- Informal care must be assessed for longevity
- Systems must intervene before collapse

What you can say:
"This arrangement relies on unpaid care that is no longer sustainable."

## OBLIGATION: SAFEGUARDING WHEN RISK EMERGES

When there is abuse, delusion, or carer breakdown, safeguards must activate.

What that means:
- Safety overrides convenience
- Silence is not neutral
- Stepping back is allowed

What you can say:

"This situation has crossed into a safeguarding issue."

That phrase matters.

## WHEN BEHAVIOUR BECOMES UNSAFE

If there is aggression, delusion, or abuse:

- "I am concerned about safety for both of us. This needs to be treated as a safeguarding issue."
- "I cannot continue in an environment where I am being accused or abused."
- "What immediate steps are being taken to reduce risk?"

You do not need to justify leaving an unsafe situation. The Act is clear: safety comes first.

# THE ESCALATION LADDER
## (USE ONLY AS NEEDED)

Escalation is not failure. It is structure.

### Step 1: Provider / Clinician
- Ask for documentation
- Ask who is accountable
- Ask for a review

### Step 2: Assessment Authority (ACAT / RAS)
- Request reassessment
- Name risk and sustainability
- Reference carer exclusion

### Step 3: Health Service / Manager
- Escalate unresolved safety issues
- Request written response

### Step 4: Oversight Body
- Aged Care Quality and Safety Commission
- My Aged Care complaints pathway
- Public Guardian (for capacity/EPOA issues)

You do not have to climb the ladder all at once. Sometimes simply knowing it exists changes the conversation.

## *IF YOU NEED TO ESCALATE CALMLY*

"I'm not comfortable with how this is being managed, and I need to escalate this to ensure safety."

"Can you please tell me who the appropriate escalation contact is?"

"I'd prefer to resolve this collaboratively, but I need clarity on next steps."

This keeps doors open — while protecting you.

## *THE RIGHT TO STEP BACK*

**One of the hardest truths carers need to hear is this: You are allowed to leave when safety is gone.**

The Act does not require carers to absorb abuse. It does not require endurance without protection. It does not require sacrifice without limits.

Stepping back is not abandonment. It is a signal that the system must now step forward.

## *WHAT THIS CHAPTER WANTS YOU TO KNOW*

- Visibility is not confrontation
- Calm language is powerful
- Documentation is protection
- Escalation is a tool, not a threat
- The law is on your side — even if practice lags behind
- You do not need to shout.
- You do not need to apologise.

## *YOU DO NOT NEED TO DISAPPEAR.*

## *LOOKING AHEAD*

The next chapter will tackle one of the most confusing and emotionally charged areas for carers:

Money, payments, and the myth of "support."

Because financial stress is where many carers are quietly crushed — and where clarity is desperately needed.

But for now, hold this:

**When you make yourself visible, you are not being difficult.**

**You are making care safer.**

**And that is exactly what the new Aged Care Act intends.**

# Chapter 8

## *MONEY, PAYMENTS, AND THE MYTH OF SUPPORT*

If the aged care system truly valued carers, money would make sense.

It doesn't.

Instead, carers are handed a confusing mix of payments, fees, subsidies, co-contributions, thresholds, waiting lists, and assumptions — all wrapped in the comforting language of support.

This chapter is about pulling that language apart. Because while the system talks about support, carers often experience financial erosion. Slow. Quiet. Relentless.

The Big Myth: "At Least There's Financial Help." Yes, there is financial help.

But it is:
- limited
- conditional
- slow to access
- disconnected from real workload
- built on the assumption that carers will fill the gaps for free

Carers are rarely told upfront:

- what support actually costs
- what they are expected to absorb
- how much unpaid labour is assumed
- how quickly "help" becomes a bill

The myth isn't that support exists. The myth is that it's enough.

# CARER PAYMENTS

## WHAT THEY REALLY ARE (AND AREN'T)

Carer Payment - This is an income support payment — not a wage.

It is:
- means-tested
- tied to strict eligibility rules
- based on caring preventing you from working

It is not payment for care provided.

And it does not reflect:
- complexity of care
- hours worked
- behavioural or medical risk
- emotional toll

Many carers describe it as:

"A holding payment so you don't fall completely through the cracks."

Carer Allowance - This is a supplement.

- It does not replace income.
- It does not reflect workload.
- It does not scale with need.

It is recognition — not compensation.

## WHAT THE NEW AGED CARE ACT ASSUMES (QUIETLY)

Under the new Aged Care Act, care is meant to be:
- person-centred
- sustainable
- wellbeing-focused

But the funding model still quietly assumes:
- a carer will be present
- a carer will coordinate
- a carer will absorb unpaid labour
- a carer will manage crises

The Act recognises carers in principle. The funding still relies on them in practice.

## HOME CARE PACKAGES

## SUPPORT WITH A PRICE TAG

Home Care Packages are often described as government-funded support. What carers discover is:
- the package belongs to the person, not the carer
- administration fees reduce actual care hours
- services often cost more than expected
- when funds run out, care doesn't stop — carers step in

A package may look generous on paper. In reality, carers are often still:
- managing nights
- handling behaviours
- coordinating appointments
- providing supervision that isn't "billable"

The system funds tasks. Carers provide continuity.

## THE HIDDEN COSTS CARERS ABSORB

Most carers don't track what they spend. If they did, the numbers would be shocking.

Hidden costs include:
- reduced work hours or lost careers
- superannuation loss
- increased health costs
- transport
- home modifications
- private services during waiting periods

None of these appear in care plans. All of them affect wellbeing.

## WHY MONEY CONVERSATIONS
## FEEL SO UNCOMFORTABLE

Carers are often reluctant to talk about money because:

- it feels selfish
- it feels transactional
- it feels like putting a price on love

The system benefits from that discomfort.

Under the new Act, sustainability matters — and sustainability includes finances. If care costs you your health, your income, and your future security, it is not sustainable.

## THE MOMENT CARERS BREAK FINANCIALLY

For many carers, the breaking point isn't emotional. It's financial.

- savings run out
- bills stack up
- employment becomes impossible
- choices narrow

By the time money becomes visible, damage is already done.

**This chapter exists to say:**
You are not bad with money. The system is designed this way.

## MAPPING THIS TO THE NEW AGED CARE ACT
## OBLIGATION: SUSTAINABLE CARE

Care arrangements must be sustainable — not propped up by financial self-harm.

Reality:
Financial strain is rarely assessed.

Carer language that matters:

"This care arrangement is no longer financially sustainable."

That sentence carries weight.

## *OBLIGATION: CARER WELLBEING*

Wellbeing includes economic security.

Reality:
Carer poverty is treated as collateral damage.

What carers are allowed to say:

"Continuing at this level is causing financial harm."

Obligation: Transparency

People are entitled to understand costs, fees, and contributions.

Reality:
Complexity hides burden.

What carers can ask:

"Can you show me what support actually looks like once fees are deducted?"

# SCRIPT CARDS

These are designed to be used verbatim. No explaining. No justifying. No apologising.

## WHEN MONEY IS TIGHT
"I need to talk about whether this care arrangement is financially sustainable."

## WHEN SERVICES ASSUME YOU'LL FILL THE GAP
"Those hours aren't covered. Who is responsible for the remaining care?"

## WHEN YOU'RE TOLD 'THAT'S JUST HOW IT IS'
"If that's the case, I need this documented as an unfunded care gap."

## WHEN FEES EAT INTO CARE
"Can you explain how much of this package actually goes to care?"

## WHEN YOU'RE EXPECTED TO WORK MORE FOR FREE
"I'm being asked to absorb unpaid care that affects my income and health."

## WHEN YOU NEED TO SAY NO
"I can't continue providing this level of unpaid care."

## WHEN YOU NEED ESCALATION

"This has become a financial sustainability issue. What are the next steps?"

## WHEN GUILT CREEPS IN

"Needing financial support does not mean I care less."

## WHAT THIS CHAPTER WANTS YOU TO KNOW

- Financial strain is a system issue, not a personal failure
- Payments are not wages
- Packages do not replace carers
- Sustainability includes money
- You are allowed to name financial harm

Carers don't fail because they ask about money. They fail when money is ignored.

## LOOKING AHEAD

The next chapter moves back into daily reality: Care at home — the parts no brochure prepares you for:
Dementia.
Incontinence.
Sleep deprivation.
Safety.
The grind.
Because understanding money helps — but understanding what it costs to live this life matters even more.

# Chapter 9

## CARE AT HOME

### THE PARTS NO BROCHURE PREPARES YOU FOR

No one tells you this part.

They talk about support.
They talk about independence.
They talk about ageing at home as though it's a gentle, dignified glide into later life.

They do not talk about:
- the nights without sleep
- the constant vigilance
- the bodily work
- the erosion of privacy
- the way your world slowly shrinks

This chapter is not here to scare you.

It's here to tell the truth — so you stop wondering why this feels so much harder than you expected.

## DEMENTIA

## WHEN THE RULES OF REALITY CHANGE

Dementia doesn't arrive all at once. It slips in quietly.

- A forgotten appointment
- A misplaced item
- A repeated story

At first, you adjust. Then the rules change.

- Logic stops working.
- Reassurance stops reassuring.
- Arguments go in circles and come back louder.

You learn — painfully — that you cannot reason someone out of a reality they didn't reason themselves into.

And yet, carers keep trying. Because love makes you hope.

## THE EMOTIONAL WHIPLASH

One moment, they are lucid and kind. The next, suspicious, angry, or frightened.

You become:
- a target for fear
- a stand-in for loss
- the face of everything that's wrong

This is one of the cruellest parts of dementia care. You are doing your best — and being blamed anyway.

## WHAT NO ONE PREPARES YOU FOR

Dementia can bring:
- paranoia
- delusions
- accusations
- emotional volatility
- loss of empathy

Being accused of harm by someone you are sacrificing everything for is devastating. It is also, tragically, not uncommon. This is not a failure of care. It is a symptom of disease.

## DEMENTIA, DELUSIONS AND CAPACITY

## THE TRUTH MOST CARERS AREN'T TOLD

First, the most important principle - Capacity is not all-or-nothing. But delusions can absolutely negate capacity for specific decisions. This is not controversial in law or medicine — it's just often ignored in practice.

**What "capacity" actually means (in real terms)**
In Australia, decision-making capacity generally requires that a person can:
- Understand the relevant information
- Retain that information long enough to make a decision
- Use or weigh that information to reach a decision
- Communicate their decision

This is called decision-specific capacity. A person may have capacity for:
- choosing what to eat
- deciding what to wear

But not have capacity for:
- medical treatment decisions
- care arrangements
- appointing or revoking an EPOA

Where delusions change everything.
A delusion is not:
- a preference
- a personality trait
- stubbornness
- anger
- disagreement

A delusion is:
- a fixed false belief that is not amenable to reason or evidence.

When delusions are present, they directly affect Step 3 above:
- the ability to use or weigh information.

That is the critical point.

**When delusions negate capacity (plain English)**
A delusion negates capacity when it directly informs the decision being made.

Examples:
- Believing a carer is trying to kill them
- Believing staff are poisoning food
- Believing money is being stolen when it isn't
- Believing they are being imprisoned or controlled

In these situations:
- the person cannot objectively weigh risk
- decisions are based on fear, not reality
- consent or refusal is not truly informed

At that point, capacity for care and safety decisions is compromised.

# THE MISTAKE SYSTEMS OFTEN MAKE

Many professionals confuse:
- ability to speak clearly

with
- capacity to decide safely

A person can:
- sound articulate
- express strong opinions
- appear assertive

And still lack capacity — if those opinions are driven by delusions.

**Clarity of speech ≠ clarity of reasoning.**

**Dementia + delusions = a safeguarding trigger**

**Under best practice (and aligned with the new Aged Care Act):**

When a person with dementia:
- develops delusions
- makes serious allegations
- refuses care based on false beliefs

This should automatically trigger:
- capacity reassessment
- safeguarding review
- involvement of substitute decision-makers (EPOA / Guardian)

It should not trigger:
- exclusion of carers
- unquestioned acceptance of allegations
- informal revocation of legal authority

## SUPPORTED DECISION-MAKING HAS LIMITS (THIS MATTERS)

The new Aged Care Act emphasises supported decision-making — but this is widely misunderstood. Supported decision-making applies:
- only while capacity exists
- only where beliefs are reality-based

It does not apply when:
- decisions are driven by delusions
- paranoia distorts risk perception
- the person cannot weigh consequences

At that point:
- substitute decision-making is not a failure — it is a safeguard.

**The key test carers can remember**
Here is a simple, powerful question:
"Is this decision being made on accurate information, or on a false belief?"

If the answer is false belief — capacity is impaired for that decision.

**Why this matters for carers**
Carers are often told:
"She knows what she wants"
"He's allowed to make bad choices"
"We have to respect autonomy"

Those statements are only true if capacity exists.

Respecting autonomy does not mean:
- abandoning someone to delusions
- exposing carers to harm
- ignoring medical evidence

**That is not autonomy. That is neglect disguised as respect.**

**Why carers are often the first to notice**

Carers see:

- patterns
- inconsistencies
- escalation
- paranoia that only appears at home

Professionals see snapshots.

This is why carer input is critical in capacity assessments — and why excluding carers leads to unsafe decisions.

**What carers are allowed to say (and should say)**

Here are phrases that are clinically and legally accurate:

- "These decisions are being driven by delusional beliefs."
- 
- "She cannot weigh information accurately because of paranoia."
- 
- "This is a capacity issue, not a preference issue."
- 
- "Supported decision-making is no longer appropriate here."

These are not emotional statements. They are capacity statements.

A hard but important truth!

A person can:

- look calm
- sound convincing
- insist strongly

And still lack capacity. Dementia is not always obvious. Delusions often appear before memory loss becomes profound. By the time systems accept loss of capacity, carers have often been living in danger for months.

# *INCONTINENCE*

## *THE WORK NO ONE TALKS ABOUT*

Incontinence strips away dignity — for everyone involved.

It is:
- constant
- unpredictable
- physically demanding
- emotionally draining

You learn to:
- read subtle cues
- clean without shaming
- manage laundry that never ends
- carry wipes, pads, spare clothes everywhere

You also learn how isolating this work is — because people don't talk about it. Yet it shapes your days and nights more than almost anything else.

## *THE TOLL ON THE CARER*

Incontinence care is:
- repetitive
- intimate
- relentless

It requires physical strength, emotional restraint, and constant attention.
Carers develop back injuries. They lose sleep. They lose patience — and then feel guilty for it.
None of this means you are unkind. It means you are human.

## SLEEP DEPRIVATION

## THE QUIET DESTROYER

Sleep loss doesn't announce itself dramatically. It accumulates. You wake for:

- toileting
- wandering
- anxiety
- pain
- confusion

You sleep lightly — always listening. Over time:

- your thinking slows
- your tolerance shrinks
- your emotions flatten or explode

Sleep deprivation makes everything harder:

- decisions
- patience
- advocacy
- safety

It is one of the biggest predictors of carer burnout — and one of the least addressed.

## SAFETY - LIVING ON HIGH ALERT

Caring at home turns you into a risk manager. You scan constantly for:

- falls
- wandering
- stove use
- medication errors
- unsafe behaviours

Your home stops feeling like a place of rest. It becomes a monitored environment. And you are the alarm system.

## *WHEN SAFETY STARTS TO SLIP*

There comes a point — often quietly — when you realise:

"I can't keep them safe anymore."

That realisation is terrifying. It is also responsible.

Home is not always the safest place — no matter how much love is in it.

## *THE GRIND*

### *THE PART THAT BREAKS PEOPLE*

The hardest part of caring isn't one big crisis. It's the relentlessness.

The same tasks.
The same explanations.
The same messes.
The same vigilance.

Day after day.

No weekends.
No sick leave.
No mental break.

This is where carers disappear — not because they don't care, but because they are exhausted beyond words.

## *WHY THE SYSTEM UNDERESTIMATES THIS WORK*

Care at home is often framed as:
- cheaper
- preferable
- less intensive

That framing ignores reality.
Home care shifts labour:
- from systems to individuals
- from paid workers to unpaid carers
- from visible settings to private homes

The work doesn't reduce. It just becomes invisible.

## *WHAT THIS CHAPTER WANTS YOU TO KNOW*

If you are:
- exhausted
- short-tempered
- grieving someone who is still alive
- wondering how much longer you can do this

You are not failing.

You are responding to an extraordinarily demanding reality.

There is no prize for enduring longer than is safe.

## *A HARD TRUTH - (SAID GENTLY)*

Love does not make care sustainable.

It makes it meaningful — but not limitless.

There comes a point where:
- support is insufficient
- risk outweighs intention
- and something has to change

Recognising that moment is not giving up. It is paying attention.


## *LOOKING AHEAD*

The next chapter tackles one of the hardest decisions carers face:

When home is no longer safe — and how to know when you've reached that point.

Not as failure.

Not as betrayal.

But as a shift — necessary, painful, and sometimes lifesaving.

Because caring is not about holding on at all costs. It is about choosing the safest possible care — for everyone involved.

# Chapter 10

## *WHEN HOME IS NO LONGER SAFE*

### *AND HOW TO KNOW YOU'VE REACHED THAT POINT*

There is a moment carers rarely talk about. Not because it doesn't happen — but because it feels like saying it out loud might make it true. It's the moment you realise that love, effort and good intentions are no longer enough to keep someone safe at home.

This chapter is about that moment.
Not as failure.
Not as betrayal.
But as a shift — necessary, painful, and sometimes lifesaving.

### *WHY THIS IS THE HARDEST CHAPTER FOR CARERS*

Carers are taught — explicitly and implicitly — that holding on is the measure of success. Staying longer. Trying harder. Managing more. So when home begins to feel unsafe, carers often turn the blame inward.

"If I were stronger…"
"If I were more patient…"
"If I just tried one more thing…"

But home does not become unsafe because carers stop caring. Home becomes unsafe because needs outgrow what one person — or one environment — can provide.

## THE MYTH THAT HOME IS ALWAYS BEST

"Aging at home" is presented as the gold standard. And often, it is. But the truth is quieter and more complicated: Home is only best while it is safe. Once safety erodes, staying at home can become:
- dangerous
- isolating
- traumatic
- medically risky

The system is slow to admit this. Carers usually realise it first.


## HOW THE SHIFT HAPPENS (USUALLY QUIETLY)

Home rarely becomes unsafe all at once. It happens in increments.

A fall that almost happened.
A night you didn't sleep at all.
A medication mistake you caught just in time.
An accusation that shook you to the core.
A moment when you realised you were afraid.


Carers often describe it as: "Something tipping." Nothing dramatic. Just unmistakable.

## THE SAFETY MARKERS CARERS RECOGNISE BEFORE ANYONE ELSE

You may have reached this point if:
- You cannot leave the house without anxiety
- Nights are more dangerous than days
- Delusions or aggression are escalating
- You are being accused, threatened, or abused
- You are physically unable to manage care tasks
- Your own health is deteriorating
- You are constantly preventing disasters
- You feel relief at the idea of someone else taking over

Relief is not a betrayal. It is information.


## WHEN LOVE IS NO LONGER THE LIMITING FACTOR

This is a hard truth, but an important one:

Love does not make care safe.
Love does not prevent falls.
Love does not neutralise dementia.
Love does not replace supervision.

Love sustains you — but it does not replace infrastructure. When carers are told "If you loved them, you'd keep them home", harm follows.

That narrative needs to stop.

## THE MOMENT CARERS RARELY ADMIT

Many carers reach a point where they think:

"If I keep doing this, someone will get seriously hurt — and it might be me."

That is not abandonment. That is risk awareness.
And risk awareness is the foundation of responsible care.


## WHY STAYING TOO LONG CAN CAUSE LASTING HARM

Carers who push past this point often experience:
- trauma
- injury
- long-term health consequences
- fractured relationships
- deep resentment
- guilt that doesn't disappear

Sometimes the greatest harm comes not from leaving —but from staying too long.

## THE SYSTEM'S QUIET RELIANCE ON DELAY

The system often delays intervention because:
- carers are still coping enough
- crisis hasn't formally occurred
- services are stretched
- waiting lists exist

Carers fill the gap. Until they can't. Then the shift is sudden and chaotic — when it could have been planned and supported.

## WHAT THE NEW AGED CARE ACT RECOGNISES
## (EVEN IF PRACTICE LAGS)

Under the new Aged Care Act:
- care must be safe and sustainable
- carer wellbeing matters
- informal care is not infinite
- safeguarding overrides convenience

This means:
Recognising the limit is not failure — it is compliance.

When home is no longer safe, stepping back is not giving up.

It is activating the system's responsibility.

## *HOW TO KNOW YOU'RE ALLOWED TO STEP BACK*

You are allowed to step back when:
- safety is compromised
- capacity is impaired
- abuse is present
- supervision needs exceed your ability
- care depends on you never resting

You do not need permission to protect yourself.

You need support — and if support is absent, stepping back is a legitimate response.


## *WHAT THIS SHIFT OFTEN LOOKS LIKE IN PRACTICE*

The shift may involve:
- residential care
- respite that becomes permanent
- hospital admission followed by placement
- guardianship involvement
- increased formal care replacing informal care

None of these erase love.

They redistribute responsibility.

## *GRIEF COMES WITH THE SHIFT*
## *AND THAT'S NORMAL*

Even when the decision is right, grief follows.

You grieve:
- the life you imagined
- the role you held
- the home that once felt safe
- the promise you made quietly to yourself

Grief does not mean you chose wrong.

It means the decision mattered.


## *WHAT CARERS NEED TO HEAR (BUT RARELY DO)*

You did not fail. You adapted — again and again — until adaptation was no longer safe.

That is not weakness. That is discernment.

If you are reading this chapter and thinking: "I think I'm there." Pause. Breathe.

You are not alone.
You are not heartless.
You are not abandoning anyone.

You are recognising reality.

## THE REFRAME THAT CHANGES EVERYTHING

This is not:
- giving up
- walking away
- breaking a promise

This is:
- choosing safety
- protecting dignity
- preventing harm
- letting care evolve

Care changes shape over time. That is not failure. That is life.


## WHEN THEY SAY NO AND YOU STILL HAVE TO ACT

First, the most important truth - A person does not have the right to make an unsafe decision if they lack capacity to understand the risk. Refusal only carries legal and ethical weight if capacity exists for that decision. This is where everything turns.

### Step 1: Is This a Preference — or a Capacity Issue?
A refusal can mean very different things. A refusal with capacity looks like:
- Understanding the risks
- Acknowledging consequences
- Making a values-based choice
- Being able to explain reasoning

Example: "I know I might fall, but I accept that risk because home matters most to me."
A refusal without capacity often looks like:
- Driven by delusions or paranoia
- Denial of obvious risks
- Inability to weigh consequences
- Refusal based on false beliefs

Example:

"You're trying to lock me up."

"Everyone is poisoning me."

"I don't need help — nothing is wrong."

In the second case, refusal does not equal capacity.

**Step 2: Dementia Changes the Rules (Quietly but Completely)**

When dementia is present — especially with delusions — "refusal" must be treated as a clinical red flag, not the end of the conversation. Under best practice and aligned with the new Aged Care Act:

- refusal triggered by cognitive impairment requires reassessment
- safeguarding obligations activate
- substitute decision-making may be required

Autonomy does not override safety when capacity is impaired.

**Step 3: The Carer's Position (This Matters)**

Here is something carers are rarely told clearly enough: You cannot be required to continue providing care in an unsafe environment. If the person refuses to leave and the situation is unsafe:

- the care arrangement has already failed
- responsibility must shift to the system
- carers are allowed to step back

Staying does not make the refusal legitimate. It only hides the risk.

**Step 4: What Happens If the Person Still Refuses?**

There are four legitimate pathways — and none of them require you to force or coerce the person yourself.

**1. Capacity Reassessment**

This is the first and most important step.

Refusal should trigger:

- urgent medical review
- formal capacity assessment
- documentation of delusions or impaired reasoning

Without this, systems often default incorrectly to "choice".

## 2. Activation of the EPOA or Guardian
If capacity is impaired:
- an invoked EPOA has authority
- or a Public Guardian may need to be appointed

This allows decisions to be made in the person's best interests, even if they object. This is not punishment. It is protection.

## 3. Safeguarding / Risk Escalation
If there is:
- self-neglect
- abuse
- delusions
- carer harm
- imminent risk

Safeguarding pathways should be activated. This may involve:
- ACAT escalation
- hospital admission
- community mental health
- guardianship services

## 4. Hospital as a Turning Point (Not a Failure)
Sometimes refusal cannot be resolved at home.

Hospital admission — even short-term — can:
- stabilise cognition
- allow reassessment
- create a safer transition point

Many placements happen after hospitalisation, not before. This is not trickery. It is often the only safe pause available.

## WHAT CARERS SHOULD NOT BE ASKED TO DO

You should never be expected to:
- physically force the person to leave
- tolerate abuse or delusional accusations
- manage escalating risk alone
- "convince" someone whose reasoning is impaired
- stay to prove refusal is genuine

That is not care. That is abandonment of responsibility by the system.


## WHAT CARERS ARE ALLOWED TO SAY
## (AND SHOULD SAY)

These phrases are clinically and legally accurate:

"This refusal is driven by impaired cognition, not informed choice."

"I cannot continue caring safely in this environment."

"This situation requires capacity reassessment and safeguarding."

"I am stepping back because the risk is no longer manageable."

You do not need to justify beyond that.

## THE HARDEST PART

## (SAID GENTLY)

A person may be angry. They may feel betrayed. They may never fully understand the decision. That is heartbreaking.

But understanding is not the test. Safety is.
Many carers carry guilt because the person "didn't agree".

But agreement is not required when capacity is lost.


## WHY THIS IS NOT BETRAYAL

Betrayal is abandoning someone to danger.

Protection sometimes looks like:
- making decisions they don't want
- tolerating anger
- being misunderstood
- choosing safety over comfort

That is not cruelty. That is love expressed through responsibility.

## *IF YOU ARE STANDING IN THIS MOMENT*
## *RIGHT NOW*

If you are here — facing refusal — and feel trapped:

Please hear this clearly:
- You are not failing
- You are not heartless
- You are not overreacting
- You are at the point where care must change form.
- And you do not have to carry that alone.

## *LOOKING AHEAD*

The next chapter will focus on:

Living with the decision — guilt, grief, relief, and rebuilding life after care changes.
Because the story doesn't end when home care ends.
It transforms.
And carers deserve support through that transformation too.

# Chapter 11

## *OUT-OF-HOME CARE*

### *WHAT THE OPTIONS REALLY ARE,*
### *AND HOW TO ACCESS THEM*

When carers begin to accept that home may no longer be safe, the next feeling is often panic.

What now?
Where do we go?
How does this even work?

The system does not answer these questions clearly. Instead, carers are handed brochures, acronyms, waiting lists, and reassurances that feel disconnected from the urgency of the moment.

This chapter is about demystifying out-of-home care — not to push you toward it, but to help you understand what exists and how to access it without crisis driving every decision.

### *FIRST: OUT-OF-HOME CARE IS NOT ONE THING*

Out-of-home care is often spoken about as if it means only one outcome: "a nursing home."

In reality, it exists on a spectrum. Understanding that spectrum gives carers choice, timing, and leverage.

## OPTION 1

## *RESPITE CARE (PLANNED OR EMERGENCY)*

Respite is often the first step — and sometimes the turning point.

What it is:
- Short-term residential care
- Can be planned or accessed urgently
- Intended to give carers a break, but often used to assess longer-term needs

What carers need to know:
- Respite can last days or weeks
- It can be repeated
- It does not lock you into permanent placement
- Respite is not failure.
- It is often the safest pause available.

How to access:
- Through My Aged Care
- Requires ACAT approval
- Can be arranged quickly if risk is documented

## OPTION 2

### TRANSITIONAL OR TEMPORARY RESIDENTIAL CARE

Sometimes care shifts after:
- hospital admission
- acute illness
- sudden cognitive decline

Transitional care allows:
- stabilisation
- reassessment
- planning without immediate permanence

This option is often under-explained but can be critical when home care collapses suddenly.

## OPTION 3

### PERMANENT RESIDENTIAL AGED CARE

This is the option carers fear most — often because of guilt, stigma, and outdated perceptions. Modern residential care varies enormously. What it can provide:
- 24/7 supervision
- medication management
- personal care
- behavioural support
- safety overnight

What it does not automatically provide:
- emotional continuity
- personalised routines
- perfect staffing

Residential care is not perfect. But for some people, it is safer than home — and safety matters.

# OPTION 4

## *SPECIALIST DEMENTIA CARE*

For people with:
- significant behavioural symptoms
- wandering
- aggression
- delusions

Specialist dementia units may be more appropriate than standard residential care. Carers are often not told these exist — or are told too late. Asking explicitly matters.

# OPTION 5

## *GUARDIANSHIP-SUPPORTED PLACEMENT*

When capacity is impaired and decisions are contested, placement may occur with:
- an invoked EPOA
- a Public Guardian
- a tribunal order

This pathway is emotionally heavy — but sometimes necessary when:
- the person refuses care
- risk is high
- carers can no longer be involved safely

This is not punishment. It is a legal safeguard.

# HOW TO ACCESS OUT-OF-HOME CARE
## (STEP BY STEP)

### Step 1: ACAT Assessment (or Reassessment)
Out-of-home care requires ACAT approval.
If circumstances have changed:
- request a reassessment
- document safety risks
- emphasise sustainability and carer wellbeing

Key language that matters:
"The current care arrangement is no longer safe or sustainable."

### Step 2: My Aged Care Referral
My Aged Care coordinates:
- referrals
- approvals
- provider listings

This system can feel slow — but urgency increases when:
- risk is documented
- carers step back
- hospital is involved

### Step 3: Visiting and Choosing Services
Carers are often told to "shop around" — when they are exhausted.
Focus on:
- safety
- staffing overnight
- dementia experience
- communication practices

You are not choosing perfection. You are choosing risk reduction.

**Step 4: Financial Assessment**

Residential care involves:

- means testing
- daily fees
- accommodation payments

This process is confusing and stressful.

It is okay to:

- ask for help
- seek financial counselling
- take time where possible

No one expects carers to understand this immediately.

## *A REALITY CHECK*

## *(SAID GENTLY)*

Most out-of-home care transitions happen:

- during crisis
- after hospitalisation
- when carers are already depleted

This is not because carers waited too long.

It is because systems are reactive.

Planning earlier — even tentatively — gives carers options.

## *WHAT THIS CHAPTER WANTS YOU TO KNOW*

Out-of-home care is not abandonment
Respite is not a trick — it's a tool
Residential care is not one uniform experience
Guardianship is sometimes protective, not punitive
Access improves when carers name risk clearly

You are allowed to ask:
- What happens if I can't do this anymore?
- What options exist beyond home?
- Those are responsible questions.

The Emotional Undercurrent (Because It Matters)
Even when the decision is right, carers often feel:
- grief
- guilt
- relief
- disorientation

These emotions can coexist.

Relief does not cancel love.
Grief does not mean regret.

## LOOKING AHEAD

The next chapter will explain Government support and the new funding regime.

# Chapter 12

*GOVERNMENT SUPPORT & THE NEW FUNDING REGIME*

*WHAT'S CHANGED, WHAT HASN'T & WHAT CARERS NEED TO KNOW*

At some point in caring, most people ask the same question: "Surely the government helps more than this?"

The answer is complicated. There is government support. There is funding. And under the new Aged Care Act, there is a genuine attempt to improve fairness, safety, and accountability.

But there are also limits — structural, financial, and practical — that carers are rarely told about upfront. This chapter is about understanding the new funding regime clearly, so carers can plan, advocate, and make decisions without being blindsided.

**First: What the Government Is Actually Responsible For**

Under the new Aged Care Act, the Australian Government has clarified its role. It is responsible for:
- funding aged care services
- regulating quality and safety
- setting eligibility and assessment frameworks
- protecting the rights of older people and carers

It is not responsible for:
- providing unlimited care
- replacing family or informal support
- removing all financial contribution from individuals

This distinction matters — because many carer frustrations come from expecting the system to do something it was never designed to do.

## THE SHIFT TO A RIGHTS-BASED SYSTEM

The new Aged Care Act moves aged care away from a welfare model and toward a rights-based framework.

In principle, this means:
- care must be safe and dignified
- services must be appropriate and sustainable
- decisions must consider wellbeing
- carers must be recognised

This is a significant improvement. But rights do not automatically create resources.

They create obligations — and carers still need to ensure those obligations are acted on.


## THE NEW FUNDING REGIME: THE BIG PICTURE

The funding system is being redesigned to:
- be more transparent
- reduce inequity
- better match funding to need
- improve accountability of providers

However, at its core, the system still relies on shared funding:
- the government contributes
- the individual contributes
- carers continue to contribute unpaid labour

This has not fundamentally changed.

## SUPPORT AT HOME: THE NEW MODEL

The old system of:
- Home Care Packages
- Commonwealth Home Support Program

is being replaced by a single Support at Home program.

What this is meant to improve:
- simpler access
- clearer funding
- less fragmentation
- quicker response to changing needs

What carers should know:
- support will still be capped
- care hours will still be finite
- administration costs will still exist
- informal care is still assumed

This is not unlimited home care.

It is structured support within limits.

## RESIDENTIAL AGED CARE FUNDING

Residential care remains:
- heavily subsidised
- means-tested
- contribution-based

Government funding covers:
- care
- clinical needs
- staffing requirements

Individuals may still pay:
- daily fees
- accommodation costs
- additional service fees

The new regime improves transparency — but not affordability for everyone.

This is a reality carers need to plan for early.


## WHAT HAS IMPROVED FOR CARERS

Under the new Act:
- carer wellbeing is explicitly recognised
- sustainability of care matters
- safeguarding obligations are clearer
- exclusion of carers is harder to justify

Carers now have stronger language to say:
"This arrangement is not compliant because it is not sustainable." That matters.

## WHAT HAS NOT CHANGED

## (AND PROBABLY WON'T SOON)

Some things remain stubbornly the same:
- carers are still unpaid
- waiting lists still exist
- services are still stretched
- crisis still accelerates access
- emotional labour remains invisible

The system is improving — but it is not generous.


## WHY FUNDING STILL FEELS LIKE A MAZE

Funding feels confusing because it is:
- layered
- conditional
- income-tested
- needs-based
- service-dependent

Carers often feel they are missing something.

Usually, they aren't.

The system really is that complex.

## WHAT CARERS SHOULD DO WITH THIS INFORMATION

Instead of trying to "master" the system, carers are better served by:
- understanding the limits
- naming sustainability issues early
- planning for transitions before crisis
- asking for reassessments when needs change
- documenting financial and emotional strain

Clarity beats optimism.


## A GENTLE BUT HONEST REMINDER

Government support is a framework, not a safety net.

It works best when:
- carers are visible
- risks are named
- limits are respected
- care changes form when needed

It works worst when carers quietly absorb what the system cannot provide.

## WHAT THIS CHAPTER WANTS YOU TO KNOW

The new funding regime improves fairness, not abundance.

Rights create leverage, not automatic solutions.

Carers still matter to system functioning.

Sustainability is now a legitimate argument.

You are allowed to plan beyond home care.

Understanding funding is not about becoming cynical.

It is about becoming informed.

## LOOKING AHEAD

The next chapter looks at how to choose an aged care facility (nursing home).

# Chapter 13

## *CHOOSING AN AGED CARE FACILITY*

### *LOOKING BEYOND THE BROCHURE*

Choosing an aged care facility is one of the most emotionally loaded decisions carers ever make. By the time you reach this point, you are often:
- exhausted
- grieving
- under time pressure
- afraid of choosing "wrong"

Facilities know this.

They offer reassurance, glossy brochures, and carefully curated tours — usually at the quietest time of day.

This chapter is not about fear. It's about seeing clearly.

### *FIRST: THERE IS NO PERFECT FACILITY*

Let's say this upfront, because it matters. There is no perfect nursing home.
There are:
- safer ones
- better-managed ones
- better-matched ones

Your task is not to find perfection. Your task is to reduce risk and increase dignity.

## What Actually Matters (And What Matters Less), Matters More Than You Think
- staffing consistency
- overnight supervision
- staff confidence with dementia
- communication with families
- response to behavioural changes
- medication management
- leadership stability

## Matters Less Than You Think
- fancy foyers
- fresh flowers
- gourmet menu descriptions
- spotless common areas at 10am
- buzzwords like "luxury" or "lifestyle"

A calm resident at 2am matters more than a cappuccino machine.

## Start With Needs, Not Location
Carers often begin with: "What's nearby?"
A better first question is: "What level of care is actually required now — and likely soon?"

Consider:
- dementia progression
- mobility
- continence
- behavioural symptoms
- medical complexity
- need for supervision

Choosing a facility that only just meets current needs often leads to another move later. And moves are hard.

## UNDERSTANDING DIFFERENT TYPES OF FACILITIES

Not all nursing homes are the same.
Some specialise in:
- high physical care
- dementia support
- behavioural management
- palliative care

Ask explicitly:
"What types of residents do you do best with?"

If they hesitate — listen.

## THE TOUR

### WHAT TO WATCH, NOT WHAT YOU'RE SHOWN

Tours are performances. Your job is to look sideways.

**Watch the Residents**
Do they look settled or distressed?
Are they engaged or parked?
Are staff interacting — or just moving people around?

**Watch the Staff**
Do they know residents' names?
Do they speak kindly and confidently?
Do they seem rushed or supported?

**Watch the Environment**
Are doors locked appropriately for safety?
Is wandering managed calmly?
Are there quiet spaces, not just activity rooms?

# ASK THE QUESTIONS THAT ACTUALLY MATTER

**Here are questions carers are often afraid to ask — but should.**

### Staffing
"What is your staffing ratio overnight?"
"How often do residents see agency staff?"
"Who makes decisions after hours?"

### Dementia and Behaviour
"How do you respond to agitation or paranoia?"
"What is your approach to behavioural symptoms?"
"How do you involve families when behaviour changes?"

### Medical Care
"How are GPs involved?"
"How are medication changes handled?"
"When do you transfer residents to hospital?"

### Communication
"How will you keep me informed?"
"Who is my point of contact?"
"How do you handle complaints?"

Facilities that answer clearly are usually safer.

### Trust Your Unease
Carers often say: "I couldn't explain it — it just didn't feel right." That feeling matters.

Unease often picks up on:
- staff stress
- poor leadership
- high turnover
- underlying chaos

You do not need evidence to pause.

## *WHAT THE NEW AGED CARE ACT CHANGES HERE*

Under the new Aged Care Act:
- residents' rights are clearer
- quality standards are being strengthened
- safeguarding obligations are more explicit
- complaints processes are more visible

This gives carers:
- stronger grounds to ask questions
- clearer expectations of transparency
- more confidence to walk away

You are not being demanding. You are engaging with a regulated service.

## *FINANCIAL CONVERSATIONS*
## *(WITHOUT SHAME)*

Money matters — and pretending it doesn't helps no one. **Ask:**

"What are the total weekly costs?"
"What is included and what is extra?"

"How do fees change if care needs increase?"

A facility that avoids financial clarity early is unlikely to improve later.

## THE REALITY OF TIMING

Many placements happen under pressure.

If you can:
- shortlist early
- visit before crisis
- ask questions calmly

You give yourself options.

If you can't — be gentle with yourself.

Urgent decisions are not moral failures.


## WHEN THE PERSON DOESN'T WANT TO GO

Resistance is common — especially with dementia.

Remember:
- agreement is not always possible
- safety still matters
- capacity determines consent

You are choosing care, not punishing.

## RED FLAGS TO TAKE SERIOUSLY

Be cautious if:
- staff minimise behavioural concerns
- carers are excluded from discussions
- turnover is visibly high
- questions are deflected
- complaints processes are unclear

Trust patterns, not promises.

## WHAT THIS CHAPTER WANTS YOU TO KNOW

Choosing a facility is not betrayal. You are allowed to ask hard questions. You are not shopping — you are assessing risk. Feeling relief does not cancel love. Walking away is sometimes the right decision. A good facility will welcome scrutiny. A poor one will resent it.

## LOOKING AHEAD

The next chapter will focus on: Moving in, settling, and what carers need to know in the first weeks after placement. Because the decision doesn't end at the door. It changes — again.

# Chapter 14

## *THE FIRST WEEKS AFTER PLACEMENT*

### *WHAT NO ONE WARNS YOU ABOUT*

The move is done. The bags are unpacked. The paperwork is signed. The door closes behind you.

And suddenly, everything feels very quiet — or unbearably loud.

The first weeks after placement are not a relief in the way carers expect. They are a collision of emotions, practical adjustments, and unsettling questions no one prepares you for.

This chapter is about that time. Not to tidy it up. Not to rush you through it. But to tell the truth about what actually happens next.

### *THE EMOTIONAL WHIPLASH*

Many carers expect to feel relief. And often, they do — briefly. But relief rarely arrives alone. It is usually accompanied by:
- guilt
- grief
- anxiety
- second-guessing
- a strange sense of emptiness

You may feel calmer and devastated. Lighter and hollow. This does not mean the decision was wrong. It means the role you lived inside for so long has suddenly changed shape.

## THE MYTH OF "SETTLING IN"

Facilities often talk about residents "settling in" within a few weeks.

This can be misleading. Adjustment is not linear.

In the early weeks, many residents experience:
- increased confusion
- agitation or withdrawal
- anger toward family
- sleep disruption
- behavioural escalation

This is not necessarily a sign of poor care.

It is often transition stress — the nervous system reacting to change.

Carers are rarely warned about this.

## WHEN BEHAVIOUR GETS WORSE
## BEFORE IT GETS BETTER

One of the hardest things carers face is seeing a loved one appear worse after placement.

They may say:
"You abandoned me."
"I want to go home."
"You've ruined my life."

These words cut deeply. But they are not evidence that the move was wrong. They are often the voice of:
- loss
- fear
- confusion
- lack of control

Dementia, especially, amplifies this stage.

You are not required to absorb abuse to prove love.

Your Role Has Changed — And That's Disorienting

Before placement, you were:
- organiser
- protector
- advocate
- carer
- constant presence

After placement, your role shifts.

You may now be:
- visitor
- monitor
- emotional anchor
- liaison

This loss of function can feel like loss of identity.

Many carers ask quietly:
"Who am I now, if I'm not doing everything?"

This question deserves care — not dismissal.

## *WHAT TO FOCUS ON IN THE FIRST FEW WEEKS*

The early weeks are not the time to fix everything. They are the time to observe and stabilise.

Focus on:
- basic comfort
- safety
- communication pathways
- understanding routines
- identifying key staff

You are learning a new system — just as the resident is.

Build One Relationship First

You do not need to know everyone.

Identify:
- one senior nurse
- one care coordinator
- one consistent staff member

This person becomes your:
- information bridge
- early warning system
- reality check

Ask:
"Who should I speak to if I'm concerned?"

Clarity reduces anxiety.

## COMMUNICATION
## LESS IS MORE (AT FIRST)

Many carers feel compelled to:
- visit constantly
- check everything
- intervene quickly

This is understandable — but can backfire.

In the first weeks:
- give staff space to establish routines
- avoid contradicting care approaches publicly
- raise concerns calmly and privately

This is not about silence.

It is about timing.

## WHAT TO DOCUMENT (QUIETLY)

Keep your own notes. Nothing dramatic — just patterns. Note:
- sleep changes
- appetite
- mood shifts
- hygiene
- communication issues
- staff responsiveness

Documentation is not mistrust. It is protection — for everyone.

## *GUILT WILL LOOK FOR EVIDENCE*

Guilt is relentless in the early weeks.

It will whisper:

"They look sad because of me."

"If I stayed, this wouldn't be happening."

"I moved them too soon."

Guilt rarely asks fair questions. It ignores:
- the risks that existed
- the nights you didn't sleep
- the safety issues you managed alone

When guilt speaks, answer it with facts — not arguments.


## *VISITING*

## *FINDING A SUSTAINABLE RHYTHM*

There is no correct visiting schedule. But there is a sustainable one. Early on:
- short, regular visits may be better than long ones
- avoid staying through distress peaks if it escalates behaviour
- give yourself permission to leave when visits become harmful

Leaving is not abandonment.

It is boundary-setting.

## WHEN YOU NOTICE PROBLEMS

If concerns arise:
- name them early
- be specific
- avoid global statements

Instead of:
"Everything is terrible."

Try:
"I've noticed increased agitation in the afternoons. Can we talk about that?"

Facilities respond better to clarity than emotion — even justified emotion.


## THE GRIEF THAT FOLLOWS YOU HOME

Many carers are surprised by what happens after visits.

You may:
- cry in the car
- feel numb at home
- feel guilty for enjoying quiet
- feel lost without constant tasks

This is post-care grief — and it is real.

You have not lost the person entirely.

But you have lost the life you lived around them.

## *WHAT THE NEW AGED CARE ACT MEANS HERE*

Under the new Aged Care Act:
- families remain partners in care
- residents' dignity and wellbeing are central
- communication obligations are clearer
- complaints pathways are protected

You are not "interfering" by staying involved. You are exercising a recognised role.

**A Quiet Reframe (That Helps)**

Try this thought — gently:
"I didn't stop caring. I changed how I care."

That shift matters.

## *WHAT THIS CHAPTER WANTS YOU TO KNOW*

The first weeks are often the hardest.

Behavioural changes are common.

Guilt is not a reliable guide.

You are allowed to rest.

Your role still matters — just differently.

There is no gold medal for suffering longer than necessary.

## LOOKING AHEAD

The next chapter will look at: Living with the long-term reality of care — staying involved without losing yourself.

Because placement is not the end of caring.

It is the beginning of a new, often more sustainable chapter.

# Chapter 15

## *STAYING CONNECTED WITHOUT BURNING OUT*

One of the quietest fears carers carry after placement is this:
"If I step back, will I stop mattering?"

For so long, caring meant doing everything. Being everywhere. Knowing everything. Fixing everything.

When care moves into a facility, carers are often left without a map for what comes next — only an unspoken expectation to either disappear politely or keep hovering on the edge of exhaustion.

This chapter is about a third way.

Staying connected.
Staying involved.
Without burning out.

## *WHY BURNOUT CAN STILL HAPPEN AFTER PLACEMENT*

Many people assume burnout ends once hands-on care ends. It often doesn't. Instead, burnout changes shape. Carers now burn out from:
- constant vigilance
- unresolved guilt
- hyper-monitoring
- fear of "missing something"
- feeling responsible but powerless

You may no longer be lifting, cleaning, or managing nights — but emotionally, you're still on call. That matters.

## *REDEFINING YOUR ROLE (THIS IS ESSENTIAL)*

Before placement, your role was provider. After placement, your role becomes partner and protector.

That means:
- observing patterns
- advocating when needed
- maintaining emotional connection
- stepping in strategically, not constantly

You are no longer the system. You are part of it. That distinction protects you.


## *CONNECTION DOES NOT MEAN CONSTANT PRESENCE*

Many carers equate love with frequency. But presence is not measured in hours logged. Connection can look like:
- shorter, more intentional visits
- meaningful rituals (tea, music, photos)
- calm consistency rather than intensity
- leaving before exhaustion turns into resentment

You are allowed to pace yourself.

## *WHY BOUNDARIES ARE AN ACT OF CARE*

Boundaries protect:
- your health
- your relationship
- your capacity to advocate when it truly matters

Without boundaries:
- visits become draining
- communication becomes reactive
- small issues feel overwhelming

Boundaries are not withdrawal. They are sustainability.


## *LEARNING TO TRUST*

## *(WHILE STAYING ALERT)*

This is one of the hardest balances. You don't need to:
- check everything daily
- intervene at every change
- hover to prove care

But you do need to:
- notice patterns
- ask questions
- speak up when something doesn't sit right

Think rhythm, not surveillance.

## GUILT WILL TRY TO RUN THE SHOW

Guilt often says:
"If I cared more, I'd visit every day."

"If something goes wrong, it's my fault."

"I owe them everything."
Guilt is loud — but not wise.

You can love deeply and choose rest.

Those two things are not opposites.

## STAYING CONNECTED IN WAYS THAT NOURISH YOU

Some carers find connection through:
- bringing familiar items or music
- reading aloud
- hand massage or quiet presence
- sitting together without conversation

Connection doesn't have to be productive.

It just has to be real.

## WHEN TO STEP IN

## (AND WHEN TO STEP BACK)

Step in when:
- safety is compromised
- dignity is impacted
- patterns worsen
- communication breaks down
-

Step back when:
- issues are minor and settling
- staff are responding appropriately
- your presence escalates distress
- you feel depleted

Knowing the difference takes practice — and permission.

## FIRST-WEEKS' CHECKLIST

**Use this gently. Not everything needs fixing.**

**Your Wellbeing**
☐ Am I sleeping better than before placement?
☐ Have I eaten properly this week?
☐ Have I had time alone without guilt?
☐ Do I feel less constantly alert?

## The Resident
☐ Are they physically safe?
☐ Are basic needs being met (nutrition, hygiene, comfort)?
☐ Is behaviour stabilising or at least monitored?
☐ Are changes being communicated to me?

## The Facility
☐ Do I know who my key contact is?
☐ Do staff respond when I raise concerns?
☐ Is there a clear routine forming?
☐ Are concerns documented when raised?

## Your Role
☐ Am I observing patterns rather than reacting instantly?
☐ Am I allowed to leave visits before exhaustion?
☐ Am I reminding myself why this decision was made?

If most answers are "yes," you are doing enough.

## SCRIPTS FOR EARLY CONCERNS
### (USE VERBATIM)

These scripts are designed to keep communication clear, calm, and effective — without escalating unnecessarily.

### Script 1: When You're Noticing a Pattern
"I've noticed a change over the past week and wanted to check in before it becomes a bigger issue."

### Script 2: When Behaviour Seems to Be Increasing
"I'm seeing more agitation than before. Is this something you're observing as well, and how is it being managed?"

### Script 3: When You're Unsure Whether to Intervene
"Can you help me understand whether this is part of settling in, or something that needs adjustment?"

### Script 4: When Communication Feels Patchy
"I'd like to clarify how updates are shared so I know what to expect."

### Script 5: When You Need Documentation
"Can you please note this concern in the care plan so we can track it?"

### Script 6: When You're Feeling Overwhelmed
"I want to stay involved, but I also need to manage my own health. Can we agree on when you'll contact me and when I should step in?"

### Script 7: When Something Doesn't Feel Right
"I can't quite put my finger on it yet, but something feels off. I'd like us to keep an eye on this together."

Trusting your instincts does not require confrontation.


## THE LONG VIEW
## (THIS MATTERS)

Care is no longer a sprint. It's not even a marathon. It's a long companionship with change.

Staying connected without burning out means:

- accepting limits
- letting go of constant control
- allowing yourself to live alongside care — not inside it

That is not abandonment. It is adaptation.

## *WHAT THIS CHAPTER WANTS YOU TO KNOW*

You are allowed to rest.

You are still important.

You don't need to prove care through exhaustion.

Boundaries protect love.

Sustainable connection is the goal.

You did not step back because you stopped caring.

You stepped back because you cared enough to survive.

## *LOOKING AHEAD*

The next chapter will gently turn the focus toward you:

After caring — rebuilding identity, purpose, and life beyond the role.

Because carers don't just give time and energy.

They give themselves.

And they deserve themselves back.

# Chapter 16

## WHEN THE END IS NEAR

### END-OF-LIFE & PALLIATIVE CARE
### WHAT THE FINAL STAGE REALLY LOOKS LIKE

There comes a point in caring when the question quietly shifts. It is no longer: How do we manage this? It becomes: How do we make this gentle? End-of-life is not a single moment. It is a phase. Sometimes brief. Sometimes stretched over months. Often confusing. Almost always confronting. This chapter is not about giving up. It is about recognising when the goal of care changes. From cure to comfort. From intervention to dignity. And from fighting decline to accompanying it.

### RECOGNISING END STAGE WHEN THE BODY IS TIRED

No one sends a formal notice saying, "This is the final chapter." Instead, carers notice patterns. The person may:
- Sleep more than they are awake
- Eat less without distress
- Lose interest in conversation
- Withdraw from activities they once enjoyed
- Become weaker despite adequate care
- Experience recurrent infections
- Stop recovering fully from hospital admissions

In dementia, the shift can look like:
- Minimal speech
- Difficulty swallowing
- Increased frailty
- Loss of mobility
- Frequent aspiration or chest infections

In organ failure it may look like:
- Breathlessness at rest
- Fluid overload
- Repeated hospital admissions
- Increasing confusion

The common thread is this: recovery stops happening. Treatments that once worked no longer restore baseline. Carers often sense this before anyone says it aloud.

You may think: "This feels different." Trust that instinct.

## THE CONVERSATION MOST FAMILIES AVOID

At some point, someone needs to ask: Are we still trying to extend life or are we focusing on comfort?

This is not a cruel question. It is a clarifying one. Continuing aggressive treatment in the final stage can mean:
- More hospital transfers
- More invasive procedures
- More confusion
- More distress

Shifting to palliative care means:
- Symptom relief
- Pain management
- Emotional support
- Fewer hospitalisations
- Dying with comfort prioritised
- Choosing comfort is not choosing death.
- It is choosing quality over intervention.

## WHAT PALLIATIVE CARE ACTUALLY IS

Palliative care is often misunderstood. It is not "what happens in the last days." It is not "stopping everything."

Palliative care is specialised support focused on:
- Pain control
- Breathlessness management
- Anxiety relief
- Nausea control
- Emotional and spiritual support
- Family support

It can begin months before death. It can run alongside other treatments. It can be provided:
- At home
- In hospital
- In residential aged care
- In hospice

The earlier it starts, the calmer the transition often feels.


## PALLIATIVE CARE PATHWAYS - HOW IT IS ACCESSED

In Australia, palliative care can be accessed through:
- GP referral
- Hospital teams
- Community palliative care services
- Residential aged care clinical staff

If decline is accelerating, you can say: "I think we need a palliative approach review."

Those words matter. They signal a shift in goals. You are not surrendering. You are reframing.

# HOSPICE VS RESIDENTIAL PALLIATIVE CARE

Hospice care is specialised end-of-life care provided in a dedicated setting. It often offers:
- Higher staff ratios
- Specialist symptom control
- A quieter environment
- Dedicated family space

Residential aged care can also provide palliative care, especially under the new funding regime. Many facilities now support residents to die in place rather than transferring to hospital.

The difference is not moral. It is structural. Hospice may be appropriate when:
- Symptoms are complex
- Pain is difficult to manage
- Family support is limited

The environment at home or in aged care cannot meet clinical needs. Residential palliative care may be appropriate when:
- The person is settled
- Symptoms are manageable
- Continuity matters
- Transfer would cause distress
- There is no single correct pathway.

The question is always: Where will this be most peaceful?

# VOLUNTARY ASSISTED DYING

## A CAREFUL NOTE

Voluntary assisted dying is legal in most Australian states, but the laws differ. Eligibility criteria are strict. Capacity must be present. Safeguards are extensive.

This book is not a legal manual on VAD. But carers should understand:
- It requires decision-making capacity
- It cannot be requested by substitute decision-makers
- It follows a formal assessment pathway
- It is not the same as palliative sedation
- It is not the same as withdrawing treatment

If this conversation arises, seek direct medical and legal advice specific to your state.
Most importantly:
Wanting comfort, wanting relief from suffering and wanting to stop invasive treatment are not the same as requesting VAD. Clarity matters.


## WHAT THE FINAL WEEKS OF LIFE OFTEN LOOK LIKE

Carers are rarely told what to expect physically. In the final weeks, you may notice:
Reduced appetite
- Increased sleeping
- Less communication
- Long pauses between breaths
- Cool hands and feet
- Restlessness or agitation
- Hallucinations or altered awareness

These are common physiological changes. They are not signs you have failed. They are signs the body is slowing.

In the final days, there may be:
- Minimal intake
- Long periods of unconsciousness
- Irregular breathing patterns
- A "rattling" sound due to secretions - This sound is distressing for families. It is rarely distressing for the person. Knowing this reduces panic.

## DEATH IN RESIDENTIAL CARE

## WHAT HAPPENS

When death occurs in residential care:
- Staff confirm death
- The GP is notified
- Family is contacted
- Cultural or spiritual practices are honoured where possible

You are allowed to:
- Sit with the body
- Bring music
- Bring ritual
- Take your time
- There is no rush.

Despite institutional surroundings, the moment can be deeply intimate. Many carers describe it as quieter than they expected. Not peaceful in a cinematic way. But still.

## THE EMOTIONAL LANDSCAPE FOR CARERS

When death approaches, carers often feel:
- Anticipatory grief
- Relief mixed with dread
- Guilt for wanting suffering to end
- Exhaustion beyond language
- Fierce protectiveness

You may find yourself thinking:
"I don't want them to go."
"I don't want this to continue."

Both can be true.

When death finally comes, emotions are rarely singular. There may be:
- Tears
- Numbness
- Shock
- Profound quiet
- Unexpected steadiness

There is no correct reaction.

## A HARD TRUTH - SAID GENTLY

Dying is not always dramatic. Often it is gradual. Often it is a slowing. Often it is simply a body that has worked long enough. The measure of care at end-of-life is not how long someone lived.

It is whether they were:
- Comfortable
- Heard
- Protected
- Treated with dignity

If you advocated, if you showed up, if you adjusted when needed, if you shifted from cure to comfort - you did your job.

## WHAT CARERS NEED TO HEAR

You are allowed to:
- Ask whether treatment is still appropriate
- Choose comfort over intervention
- Say no to another hospital transfer
- Request palliative involvement early
- Sit quietly instead of fixing
- Step out of the room if it is too much
- Breathe

End-of-life is not a test of endurance. It is a passage. You are not required to be strong every minute of it.

## AFTER THE LAST BREATH

When the moment comes, time does something strange. It stretches. It contracts. You may watch the chest for movement that does not return. You may wait for someone to confirm what you already know. And then there is a stillness that feels almost unfamiliar.

Caring does not end at that moment. It changes again. But this time, the labour stops. The vigilance stops. The waiting stops. And what remains is love without responsibility. That is not nothing. It is everything that was underneath the work.

## WHAT THIS CHAPTER WANTS YOU TO KNOW

Recognising end stage is not giving up. Palliative care is active care. Hospice and residential pathways both have value. Voluntary assisted dying is legally complex and capacity dependent. Death often looks quieter than expected. Choosing comfort is not betrayal.

If you walked someone to the end with honesty and protection, you did not fail them. You accompanied them.

And no system, no legislation, no assessment framework can measure that. It is measured in presence.

And that is enough.

# AFTER CARING — WHO ARE YOU NOW?

There is a moment that comes after caring changes or ends — and it often arrives unexpectedly.

The house is quieter.
The phone doesn't ring as often.
Your days are no longer shaped around someone else's needs.

And suddenly, a question rises that feels both simple and unsettling:

Who am I now?

This chapter is not about reinvention.

It's about recognition.

## THE SPACE CARING LEAVES BEHIND

Caring fills space. It fills:
- time
- thought
- identity
- purpose

When that role changes — whether gradually or suddenly — it leaves a silence that can feel disorienting. Many carers expect relief. What they often feel first is emptiness. That emptiness is not a sign that you failed to move on. It's a sign that caring was central to your life — and now that centre has shifted.

## WHY THIS TRANSITION FEELS SO STRANGE

Caring is not just something you did. It's something you were. You were:
- needed
- relied upon
- consulted
- constantly alert

After caring changes, you may feel:
- unmoored
- unnecessary
- guilty for resting
- unsure what to do with yourself

This is not weakness. It is identity grief.


## THE GRIEF NO ONE NAMES

Carers often grieve quietly.

Not just the person — but:
- the role
- the meaning
- the intensity
- the sense of being essential

This grief is complicated because:
- the person may still be alive
- the care may not be fully over
- others may expect you to "move on"

But grief doesn't run on schedules. It runs on attachment.

## *WHEN PURPOSE FEELS LOST*

During caring, your purpose was clear. Afterwards, purpose can feel vague — even absent. You may wake up and wonder:

"What am I meant to be doing today?"

This question can feel frightening. But it's also an opening.

Purpose doesn't disappear. It changes shape.

## *WHY REST FEELS SO HARD*

Many carers struggle to rest even when they finally can. You may feel:
- anxious when nothing urgent is happening
- guilty enjoying quiet
- restless without a task
- undeserving of ease

This is not indulgence fatigue. It is a nervous system that has been on high alert for too long. Rest is not something you earn. It is something you relearn.

You Are Not "Going Back" to Who You Were. A common pressure carers feel is: "I should get back to my old self." But caring changes people. You may now be:
- more patient
- more tired
- more discerning
- less tolerant of nonsense
- deeply attuned to vulnerability

You don't need to erase these changes. You can integrate them.

## *REBUILDING IDENTITY GENTLY*

You don't need to answer "Who am I now?" all at once.

Start smaller.

Ask:
What do I enjoy — even a little?

What feels nourishing rather than draining?

What parts of caring taught me something valuable?

Identity returns through experience, not introspection alone.

Permission to Want Something New

Some carers feel shame for wanting:
- joy
- novelty
- freedom
- lightness

As though wanting more life somehow betrays what they gave. It doesn't.

Wanting a future does not erase the past. It honours it.

## *RELATIONSHIPS AFTER CARING*

Caring can narrow social worlds.

Afterwards, relationships may feel:
- awkward
- distant
- changed

Some people won't understand what you've lived through. Some will surprise you.

You don't need to explain yourself to everyone. Connection will rebuild — slowly, unevenly, honestly.

## *IF YOU ARE STILL CARING, BUT DIFFERENTLY*

For many carers, caring doesn't end cleanly.

You may still be:
- visiting
- advocating
- worrying
- holding emotional space

This chapter still belongs to you.

Identity can shift alongside ongoing care. You are allowed to be more than one thing at once.

## A QUIET TRUTH WORTH HOLDING

You are not behind.

You are not lost.

You are in transition.

Transitions feel uncertain because they are becoming, not failing.


## WHAT THIS CHAPTER WANTS YOU TO KNOW

It's normal to feel unsure of who you are now.

Emptiness is not failure — it's space.

Rest takes practice after long vigilance.

You don't owe anyone constant self-sacrifice.

You are allowed to build a life that includes joy.

You gave deeply.

You are allowed to receive — from life, from others, from yourself.

## *A GENTLE CLOSING REFLECTION*

Caring asked everything of you.

And you answered.

Now the question is different.

It's no longer:

"Who needs me?"

It's:

"What do I need?"

That question is not selfish.

**It is the beginning of your next chapter.**

# CONCLUSION

## YOU WERE NEVER MEANT TO DO THIS ALONE

If you have read this book from beginning to end, you have travelled a long way.

You've walked through:
- the shock of being thrown into caring
- the quiet, grinding realities no one prepares you for
- the maze of systems, assessments, and funding
- the moments where safety tipped and something had to change
- the grief of letting go — and the slow return to yourself

This book was never meant to teach you how to endure more. It was meant to remind you that endurance has limits — and that those limits matter.


## THE TRUTH THAT THREADS THROUGH EVERY CHAPTER

Caring is not one thing.
It is:
- love and exhaustion
- meaning and loss
- devotion and resentment
- tenderness and terror

The problem has never been that carers don't care enough.
The problem is that carers are asked to care in isolation, with systems that quietly assume they will absorb what the system cannot provide.

You were never meant to do this alone.

## WHAT THIS BOOK HAS BEEN SAYING ALL ALONG

From the first chapter to the last, one message keeps returning:
Care is a shared responsibility.

Not a private burden.
Not a moral test.
Not something to be borne silently.

When care is shared:
- people are safer
- carers last longer
- dignity is protected
- harm is prevented

When it is not — everyone suffers.


## THE REFRAME THAT CHANGES EVERYTHING

If there is one reframe to carry forward, it is this:

Asking for help is not failure.

Naming limits is not weakness.

Changing care is not betrayal.

Stepping back is not abandonment.

These are acts of responsibility.

And responsibility is at the heart of good care.

## WHAT YOU NOW KNOW

## (THAT YOU DIDN'T BEFORE)

You now know:
- how the system actually works — not how it's described
- when assessments fail and how to name that
- when autonomy ends and protection begins
- how to recognise when home is no longer safe
- what options exist beyond home
- how to stay connected without burning out
- how to find yourself again after caring changes

This knowledge is not abstract.

It is protective.


## FOR THE CARER READING THIS IN CRISIS

If you are reading this while:
- exhausted
- frightened
- unsure what to do next

Pause here. You do not need to solve everything today.

You only need to recognise that:
- You matter in this equation.
- Your wellbeing is not collateral damage.
- Your safety is not negotiable.
- Your voice is not optional.

## *FOR THE CARER WHO HAS ALREADY WALKED THIS PATH*

If caring has already changed or ended for you:

Your experience still matters.

The care you gave does not disappear when the role changes.

It lives in:
- the choices you made
- the dignity you protected
- the love you carried even when it hurt

You are allowed to carry that forward — without carrying the weight forever.


## *FOR THE HEALTH PROFESSIONAL*
## *WHO FOUND THEIR WAY HERE*

If you are a professional reading this book:

Thank you for staying.

Carers are not obstacles. They are not emotional noise. They are partners in care — and often the first to see risk.

Listening earlier changes outcomes later.

## WHAT COMES AFTER THE LAST PAGE

This book ends — but caring does not follow neat endings.

There will still be:
- hard days
- moments of doubt
- waves of grief
- unexpected relief

All of that is allowed. You are not required to be certain. You are only required to be human.

## A FINAL TRUTH

### (WORTH HOLDING ONTO)

You did not fail because caring was hard. Caring was hard because it asked something extraordinary of you. And you answered — again and again — until answering required change. That is not failure. That is love, expressed with courage.

If You Take Nothing Else With You, Take this: You were never meant to do this alone. and you don't have to carry it alone anymore.

Whatever comes next, you are allowed to move forward with:
- clarity
- compassion
- boundaries
- and hope — quiet, realistic, earned hope

You have already done one of the hardest things there is.

Now, you are allowed to live.

# REFERENCES & KEY SOURCES

## (AUSTRALIA – AGED CARE AND END-OF-LIFE CARE)

This book draws on lived experience, policy frameworks, clinical guidance and Australian legislation governing aged care, health care decision-making and end-of-life care. The following sources provide authoritative background and practical guidance for carers, professionals and families navigating the aged care system.

## AUSTRALIAN LEGISLATION AND POLICY

**Aged Care Act 2024 (Cth)**
Establishes a rights-based framework for aged care in Australia, including wellbeing principles, safeguarding obligations, recognition of carers and reforms to funding and service delivery.

**Aged Care Quality and Safety Commission Act 2018 (Cth)**
Provides the regulatory framework for monitoring aged care providers and managing complaints, serious incidents and quality standards.

**Aged Care Quality Standards (2019, updated under the new Act)**
Defines the standards aged care providers must meet in delivering safe, respectful and person-centred care.

**Serious Incident Response Scheme (SIRS)**
Mandatory reporting system for incidents in residential aged care including abuse, neglect, unexplained absence and inappropriate use of restraint.

# NATIONAL PROGRAMS AND GOVERNMENT SERVICES

**My Aged Care**
Australian Government gateway for aged care information, assessments and service referrals.
https://www.myagedcare.gov.au

**Aged Care Quality and Safety Commission**
Regulator responsible for provider oversight, complaints investigation and safeguarding.
https://www.agedcarequality.gov.au

**Services Australia – Carer Payments and Allowances**
Information on financial support available to unpaid carers.
https://www.servicesaustralia.gov.au

# SUPPORT AT HOME PROGRAM

## (REPLACING HOME CARE PACKAGES AND CHSP)

Australian Government reform program designed to simplify home-based aged care support.
**Health and Clinical Guidance**

**Palliative Care Australia**
National peak body providing guidance on palliative care services and policy.
https://www.palliativecare.org.au

**Australian Commission on Safety and Quality in Health Care**
Develops national safety standards for hospitals and health services, including discharge planning and end-of-life care.
https://www.safetyandquality.gov.au

**Advance Care Planning Australia**
National program supporting advance care directives and end-of-life planning.
https://www.advancecareplanning.org.au

## GUARDIANSHIP, CAPACITY AND SUBSTITUTE DECISION-MAKING

State and territory legislation governs decision-making capacity, guardianship and enduring powers of attorney. Carers should consult the relevant authority in their jurisdiction.

Key bodies include:

- Public Guardian / Public Advocate (state-based)

- Civil and Administrative Tribunals

- State Guardianship Offices

These bodies oversee substitute decision-making where capacity is impaired.

## VOLUNTARY ASSISTED DYING (AUSTRALIA)

Voluntary assisted dying legislation exists in several Australian states, including:

- Victoria
- Western Australia
- Tasmania
- South Australia
- Queensland
- New South Wales (from 2023)

Eligibility criteria, assessment processes and safeguards vary between jurisdictions. Individuals seeking information should consult state-specific health department guidance and independent legal advice.

## RESEARCH AND SYSTEM REVIEWS

Royal Commission into Aged Care Quality and Safety (2021)

Landmark inquiry examining systemic failures and recommending structural reform of Australia's aged care system.

## A FINAL NOTE

Policies, funding models and legislation in aged care continue to evolve. Carers are encouraged to verify current requirements with government services, health professionals and legal advisers where decisions involve safety, capacity or financial commitments.

The purpose of this reference section is not to replace professional advice. It is to point readers toward the frameworks that shape the system they are navigating.

# FOR HEALTH PROFESSIONALS

This section has been written to support health professionals, aged care providers, and allied services in refreshing their understanding of the new Aged Care Act and the Aged Care Code of Conduct, and in applying both consistently in day-to-day practice.

The Code of Conduct requires all aged care workers and providers to act with respect, integrity, and accountability; to deliver care in a safe, competent, and compassionate manner; to respect the dignity, autonomy, and rights of older people; and to communicate openly and effectively with care recipients, their families, and authorised decision-makers.

The new Act reinforces these obligations by embedding a rights-based framework that places the older person at the centre of decision-making, supported by transparency, proportionality, and lawful authority. Together, the Act and the Code establish clear expectations regarding informed consent, supported decision-making, documentation, escalation of concerns, and collaboration with carers and substitute decision-makers where appropriate.

This section is not intended to assign fault or criticise individual practitioners. Rather, it serves as a practical refresher — reconnecting legislative intent, professional conduct standards, and lived experience — to assist professionals in recognising their obligations, avoiding unintended breaches, and delivering care that is both legally compliant and ethically sound.

## IMPORTANT NOTE ON COMPLIANCE

Failure to meet obligations under the Aged Care Act or the Aged Care Code of Conduct may result in regulatory action, including investigation, enforceable undertakings, sanctions, or referral to professional oversight bodies.

# WHAT HEALTH PROFESSIONALS NEED TO UNDERSTAND ABOUT CARE AT HOME & THE NEW AGED CARE ACT

Most health professionals do not fail carers because they don't care.

They fail carers because they are trained to see:

- patients, not systems
- episodes, not trajectories
- compliance, not sustainability

Carers live in the spaces between appointments, rosters, and discharge summaries.

This chapter is written for professionals working in:

- hospitals
- ACAT / RAS teams
- community health
- aged care providers
- general practice

Its purpose is simple: To make the invisible visible.

# WHAT THE NEW AGED CARE ACT
## REQUIRES OF PRACTICE

The Act introduces a rights-based framework that reshapes professional responsibility. Health professionals are now expected to:

- consider carer wellbeing as part of care planning
- assess sustainability, not just functionality
- activate safeguards early
- recognise legally appointed decision-makers
- avoid defaulting responsibility back onto carers

### 1. Hospital Admission: The First Point of Failure (or Prevention)
### What Often Happens
- Carer details are recorded superficially
- Admission focuses on acute illness
- Cognitive changes are attributed to age or infection
- Informal care is assumed to resume post-discharge

### What the Act Requires
- Recognition of carers as key participants
- Early identification of decision-making capacity issues
- Planning for transitions, not just treatment
- Better Practice

### Health professionals should ask:
- Who provides care at home?
- Is this arrangement sustainable?
- Has cognition changed?
- Is there an EPOA or advance care document?

Failure to ask these questions early creates downstream risk.

## 2. Discharge Planning: Where Risk Is Most Often Exported
**Discharge is not an administrative event. It is a transfer of responsibility.**

### Common Practice Gaps
- No consultation with the primary carer
- No assessment of home safety
- No confirmation that care can continue
- No contingency planning

Act-Aligned Practice: Before discharge, professionals must consider:
- whether informal care is safe and sustainable
- whether cognitive or behavioural changes increase risk
- whether supports are in place before discharge

Discharging without consultation does not shift responsibility — it defers harm.

## 3. Cognitive Decline, Delusions, and Allegations: A Safeguarding Lens
When a person develops:
- paranoia
- delusions
- accusations against carers

This is not merely "challenging behaviour." It is a safeguarding trigger.

### What Goes Wrong
- Allegations are taken at face value
- Carer input is discounted
- Capacity is not reassessed
- Risk escalates silently

### What the Act Requires
- Supported decision-making with safeguards
- Reassessment of capacity when cognition changes
- Recognition that delusions undermine reliability of self-report

Ignoring this exposes:
- carers to harm
- patients to neglect
- professionals to risk

## 4. Assessments: Why Phone-Based Reviews Fail Complex Cases

Phone assessments rely heavily on:
- self-report
- coherence
- insight
- 

These are exactly the capacities compromised in:
- dementia
- delirium
- acute illness
- paranoia

Better Practice
- In-person assessments for cognitive complexity
- Mandatory carer input
- Explicit documentation of reliance on informal care

Assessments without carer input are structurally incomplete.

## 5. Carer Safety Is a Clinical Issue

Abuse of carers — verbal, emotional, or physical — is often minimised.

It should not be.

Under the Act:
- carer safety is part of care safety
- unsafe arrangements require intervention
- carers are permitted to step back

Expecting carers to tolerate abuse is neither ethical nor compliant.

## Reflective Practice Questions for Professionals

Use these in team meetings or supervision:

- Who is holding this care arrangement together?
- What happens if that person stops?
- Have we documented carer wellbeing and sustainability?
- Are we relying on goodwill instead of support?
- Would this plan survive scrutiny if the carer withdrew tomorrow?

If the answer is no — the plan is unsafe.

## 6. Enduring Power of Attorney: Recognition Is Not Optional

An EPOA is not a preference. It is a legal safeguard.

### Common Missteps

- Assuming EPOA only matters "later"
- Treating it as advisory rather than binding
- Informally disregarding it when conflict arises

### Correct Practice

### When an EPOA exists:

- it must be identified early
- it must be recognised once invoked
- it cannot be ignored without formal process

If concerns arise:

- capacity must be reassessed
- safeguarding or guardian pathways must activate

Informal rejection is not lawful practice.

## What an Enduring Power of Attorney actually is

An Enduring Power of Attorney (EPA/EPOA) is a legal document where a person (the principal) appoints someone they trust (the attorney) to make decisions if and when they lose decision-making capacity.

Key point:
"Enduring" means it continues after capacity is lost. It exists before incapacity. It becomes active when incapacity occurs (depending on how it's written).

## When an EPA is "held" vs "invoked" (this matters)
- Held (but not invoked) - The document is signed and valid
- The person still has capacity
- The attorney has no decision-making power yet
- The person still makes their own decisions

## Invoked

An EPA is invoked when:
- the person loses decision-making capacity, AND
- the EPA specifies that it operates upon incapacity (most do)

In practice, invocation usually requires:
- a medical opinion (GP, specialist, sometimes two doctors)
- written confirmation of incapacity
- notification to relevant parties (providers, banks, services)

Once invoked, decision-making authority legally transfers to the attorney for the relevant domains (health, personal, financial).

## How an EPA is correctly invoked (step by step)
Step 1: Capacity concern identified
- Cognitive decline, dementia, delirium, serious illness
- Concerns raised by carer, clinician, or assessor

Step 2: Capacity assessed
- Usually by a GP or specialist
- Capacity is decision-specific, not global
- Written statement is best practice

Step 3: EPA activated
- Attorney presents the EPA + medical evidence
- Services are notified

Attorney must now be consulted for decisions covered by the EPA.
**Important: Once invoked, services cannot simply "choose" not to recognise it.**

**What DOES NOT revoke or invalidate an EPA**
This is where systems often go wrong. An EPA is not revoked because:
- the person becomes angry with the attorney
- the person becomes suspicious or paranoid
- the person makes accusations during dementia
- the person says "I don't want them anymore" after losing capacity
- staff feel uncomfortable or prefer to deal directly with the person

None of those are legally sufficient.


## HOW AN EPA CAN BE LEGALLY REVOKED

**Scenario 1: Revocation by the person (only if they have capacity)**
A person can revoke their EPA only if they have decision-making capacity at the time of revocation.
This requires:
- capacity to understand what an EPA is
- capacity to understand the consequences of revoking it

Best practice:
- written revocation
- witnessed
- ideally supported by medical confirmation of capacity

If capacity is impaired, revocation is invalid.

## Scenario 2: Revocation by a tribunal or authority

If there are concerns about:

- abuse of power
- conflict of interest
- neglect
- misuse of funds

Then the EPA can be:

- suspended
- revoked
- replaced

But only by:

- a state tribunal (e.g. QCAT, VCAT, NCAT), or
- the Public Guardian / Public Trustee

This requires:

- investigation
- evidence
- due process

It cannot happen informally.

## What should happen if concerns are raised about an attorney

If someone alleges an attorney is harming or abusing the person:

**Correct process:**

- Safeguarding concern raised
- Capacity reassessed
- Interim protections put in place
- Referral to Public Guardian or tribunal if needed
- EPA reviewed formally

**Incorrect (but common) practice:**
- ignoring the EPA
- excluding the attorney
- accepting allegations at face value
- making decisions without authority

**Can someone "reassign" an EPA after incapacity?**
Short answer: No — not legally.

If a person:
- lacks capacity, and
- signs a new EPA, or
- verbally appoints someone else

That new arrangement is likely invalid.

Only a tribunal can appoint or replace a decision-maker once capacity is lost.
**Supported decision-making vs substitute decision-making (new Act confusion)**

The new Aged Care Act promotes supported decision-making — but:

Supported decision-making:
- applies while capacity exists
- does not override an invoked EPA
- does not allow professionals to bypass legal authority

Once capacity is lost: Substitute decision-making applies.

That's where the EPA sits.

This is a major point of confusion in current practice.

# *DEMENTIA, DELUSIONS*

# *AND DECISION-MAKING CAPACITY*

**Where Autonomy Ends and Safeguarding Begins**
**Key Principle**
Capacity is decision-specific — and delusions can negate capacity for particular decisions.

This is well established in law and medicine, yet frequently misunderstood in practice.

**What Capacity Requires (Clinical Reminder)**
A person has decision-making capacity for a specific decision if they can:
- Understand the relevant information
- Retain the information long enough to decide
- Use or weigh the information to reach a decision
- Communicate the decision
-

Failure at any one of these steps means capacity is impaired for that decision.
**Where Delusions Matter Clinically**
A delusion is a fixed false belief that:
- is not based in reality
- is not amenable to evidence or reassurance.

Delusions directly undermine the ability to use or weigh information. This is the step most often overlooked.

**Common Clinical Error**
Clinicians may conclude a person has capacity because they:
- speak fluently
- appear calm
- express consistent preferences
- strongly assert their wishes

This is not a capacity assessment. **Articulation ≠ insight. Assertion ≠ reasoning.**
A person can communicate clearly while reasoning is distorted by delusion.

## Examples Where Delusions Negate Capacity

Capacity for care or safety decisions is compromised when decisions are driven by beliefs such as:

- "My carer is trying to poison or kill me."
- "Staff are stealing from me."
- "Medication is a form of harm."
- "People are conspiring against me."

In these cases:

- risk cannot be weighed accurately
- consent or refusal is not informed
- reliance on expressed wishes may increase harm

This is a safeguarding issue, not a disagreement.

## Supported Decision-Making: Important Limits

The new Aged Care Act promotes supported decision-making. However, supported decision-making:

- applies only where capacity exists
- assumes beliefs are reality-based
- does not override medical evidence of incapacity

It does not apply where:

- delusions dominate reasoning
- paranoia drives refusal of care
- risk perception is fundamentally distorted

At this point:

Substitute decision-making is a protective mechanism, not a failure.

## Role of the Carer in Capacity Assessment

Carers often observe:

- behavioural changes not visible in clinic
- patterns of delusion or paranoia
- escalation of accusations or fear

Excluding carers:

- removes essential collateral history
- increases reliance on unreliable self-report
- leads to unsafe conclusions

Under the new Act, carers are recognised contributors — not optional informants.

## Red Flags Requiring Reassessment or Escalation
The following should trigger capacity reassessment and safeguarding review:

- New or escalating delusions
- Allegations against carers arising from cognitive decline
- Refusal of care based on false beliefs
- Breakdown of informal care arrangements
- Carer safety concerns

Ignoring these increases risk for:

- the patient
- the carer
- the service
- the clinician

## Enduring Power of Attorney (EPOA): Clinical Responsibilities
When an EPOA exists:

- It must be identified early
- It must be recognised once invoked
- It cannot be informally disregarded

If concerns arise about the attorney:

- capacity must be reassessed
- safeguarding processes must activate
- referral to the Public Guardian or tribunal may be required

Informal exclusion of an EPOA is not lawful practice.

## Practical Language for Clinicians

The following phrases are clinically accurate and defensible:

- "This decision appears to be driven by delusional beliefs."
- "The person is unable to weigh risk accurately due to paranoia."
- "Supported decision-making is no longer appropriate for this decision."
- "This is now a safeguarding issue."

Using this language:

- clarifies risk
- protects all parties
- aligns practice with legislation

## Reflective Practice Questions

Clinicians should routinely ask:

- Is this decision grounded in reality or false belief?
- Would I reach the same conclusion without carer input?
- If the carer withdrew today, would this plan remain safe?
- Am I prioritising expressed wishes over demonstrated capacity?

If uncertainty exists — pause and escalate.

## Why This Matters

Failure to recognise loss of capacity in the presence of delusions can lead to:

- unsafe discharges
- carer harm
- neglect masked as autonomy
- legal and ethical exposure

The new Aged Care Act was designed to prevent this exact outcome.

## Closing Reminder

Autonomy is meaningful only when decisions are informed. When dementia and delusions distort reality, protection is not paternalism — it is responsible care. **Listening to carers, reassessing capacity, and activating safeguards are not overreactions. They are best practice.**

# THE NEW AGED CARE ACT

## WHAT'S CHANGED — AND WHY IT MATTERS

A new era of aged care commenced on 1 November 2025 when both the Support at Home program and the new Aged Care Act took effect, marking the beginning of a transformed system.

The Albanese Government committed to "once-in-a-generation" aged care reform. Around 1.4 million Australians were expected to benefit from the Support at Home program by 2035, helping them remain in their homes as they age.

Australia's growing ageing population had profound implications for the economy, healthcare system and social services, particularly the aged care sector. Aged care in Australia was designed to promote the well-being, dignity and quality of life for older individuals who needed assistance, offering a spectrum of care options from in-home support to full-time residential services.

In 2024–2025 the Australian Parliament passed the Aged Care Act 2024, bringing in a new rights-based aged care framework that commenced on 1 November 2025. The reforms were described as the most significant in a generation, aimed at putting older people at the centre of care, strengthening quality standards, and improving access through a simplified system.

The centrepiece of the reform was the replacement of the old Home Care Packages Program with a new Support at Home program, also effective from 1 November 2025. This program was designed to help older Australians remain independent in their homes and communities for longer with a clearer, more flexible in-home care structure.

A "no worse off" principle was applied: people already receiving home or residential aged care continued to have at least the same level of funding and contributions as under the previous system, with protections for existing arrangements during the transition.

# KEY STATISTICS AND TRENDS

Growing Elderly Population
Australia's population has been ageing for decades. As of recent estimates, around 16 percent of Australians were aged 65 and over, with this proportion forecast to rise significantly by mid-century due to longer life expectancy and changes in demographic structure.

Longer Life Expectancy
Australians were living longer, with life expectancy estimates for people born in the early 2020s at around 82.9 years for males and 85 years for females, driven by improvements in healthcare and living standards. (These figures are consistent with recent Australian Bureau of Statistics life expectancy data.)

Baby Boomer Generation
The ageing of the large baby boomer cohort (born 1946–1964) continued to drive demand for aged care services as more people reached retirement and later ages.

# SUPPORT AT HOME PROGRAM

The Support at Home program replaced the Home Care Packages Program and Short-Term Restorative Care on 1 November 2025, meaning people who were already receiving a Home Care Package kept the same funding level and unspent funds when they transitioned to the new system. The Commonwealth Home Support Program is scheduled to transition into the Support at Home program no earlier than 1 July 2027.

The new program introduced eight funding classifications for in-home care based on need, with tailored support including home modifications and assistive technology to help people maintain independence. Support at Home was projected to help approximately 1.4 million people remain in their homes by 2035.

## System Simplicity and Equity

A Single Assessment System was introduced to simplify access and make eligibility clearer across care settings.

Existing care arrangements and contributions were protected under the no worse off principle when transitioning to the new system, ensuring people did not pay more than they would have under older arrangements.

## In-Home Support Innovations

The Support at Home program expanded access to:
home modifications
assistive technology and equipment
restorative support for recovery after illness or injury
more flexible, personalised in-home services
These changes were designed to help older Australians stay independent and connected to their communities.

## Residential Aged Care Changes

The reforms also included provisions aimed at improving funding sustainability and quality in residential aged care, with stronger quality standards and accountability mechanisms under the new Aged Care Act. Providers are now subject to clearer regulatory expectations to deliver safe, respectful, and high-quality services. The Taskforce that informed these reforms included older Australians, carers, experts and providers, and recommended updates to how aged care is funded and delivered, including clearer means-tested contributions and protections for people's homes.

The family home's treatment didn't change as part of the reforms — it continues to be exempt from aged care means testing in most cases.
Government contributions remain the majority share for aged care, with many residents continuing to have relatively low out-of-pocket contributions relative to government support.

## Rights, Regulation and Safety

The Aged Care Act 2024 established a Statement of Rights for older Australians receiving care, with a positive duty on providers to uphold these rights and stronger regulatory powers to investigate poor practice and protect people from harm.

**The reforms increased:**
transparency and accountability for providers
regulatory powers of the Aged Care Quality and Safety Commission
mechanisms for complaints, whistleblower protection, and enforcement of standards.

These reforms aimed to ensure the system was safer, more respectful and rights-centred.

**Financial Arrangements and Contributions**
Under Support at Home, the funding model was designed to be clearer and fairer, with:
government funding covering clinical care fully
contributions from individuals for other support services based on means and ability to pay
protections ensuring existing recipients did not pay more than under previous arrangements.

(Your specific percentages by pension status will vary under the new classifications issued by Services Australia and My Aged Care; up-to-date contribution tables are available on official government resources such as the Support at Home program pages on health.gov.au and myagedcare.gov.au.)

## WHY THESE REFORMS MATTER

The reforms were intended to address decades-long issues in the aged care system by:

- putting older Australians' rights at the centre
- simplifying access and eligibility
- making care more personalised and sustainable
- improving quality and safety oversight heading into the future

## *WHAT THIS MEANS IN REAL LIFE*

## *(PLAIN ENGLISH)*

The old system rationed care by package levels and long waits.

The new system aimed to match care more closely to actual need.

Clinical care is now fully funded, not something carers had to fight for.

Existing carers were protected from paying more under the transition.

Support at Home acknowledged what carers already knew: needs change, and care must change with them.

## *ONE IMPORTANT REALITY CHECK*

Even under Support at Home:

- care is still capped
- carers are still assumed to fill gaps
- funding is still not unlimited

The reform improved fairness and clarity, not abundance.

## *WHAT THIS CHAPTER*

## *ASKS OF HEALTH PROFESSIONALS*

Not perfection. Not heroics.

Just this:
- Ask one more question
- Listen to one more voice
- Pause before assuming
- Document risk clearly
- Act before crisis

**Why This Matters**
When carers disappear, systems collapse. Not because carers failed — but because they were never properly seen.

**The new Aged Care Act gives professionals permission to:**
- slow down
- share responsibility
- intervene earlier
- protect everyone involved

But only if it is translated into practice.

# GLOSSARY OF AGED CARE TERMS
## (AUSTRALIA)

The aged care system uses language that can feel technical and confusing, particularly for families encountering it for the first time. This glossary explains commonly used terms in plain language so carers can better understand how the system operates and what services are available.

**Why This Glossary Matters**
Understanding the language of aged care helps carers:
- ask informed questions
- recognise their rights
- navigate assessments and services
- advocate effectively for the person they care for

**ACAT / ACAS (Aged Care Assessment Team / Aged Care Assessment Service)**
A multidisciplinary team that assesses whether an older person is eligible for higher-level aged care services. This assessment is required before someone can receive a Home Care Package or enter residential aged care.

**Advance Care Directive**
A written document that records a person's preferences for future health care if they lose decision-making capacity. It may include wishes about life-sustaining treatment, palliative care and other medical decisions. Names and legal requirements vary between states.

**Aged Care Quality and Safety Commission**
The independent national regulator responsible for monitoring aged care providers, managing complaints and ensuring services meet the Aged Care Quality Standards.

**Aged Care Quality Standards**
National standards that all government-funded aged care providers must meet. They focus on dignity, safety, quality of care, governance and the rights of older people receiving services.

## Behaviour Support Plan

A structured plan used when an older person displays behaviours that may put themselves or others at risk. It outlines strategies to reduce distress and prevent the inappropriate use of restrictive practices.

## Carer

A person who provides ongoing support to someone with illness, disability or frailty. Most carers are family members, partners or close friends and provide care without payment.

## Carer Allowance

A fortnightly payment from Services Australia available to people providing daily care to someone with a disability or medical condition.

## Carer Payment

An income support payment for people who cannot participate in full-time work because they provide constant care to someone with severe disability, illness or frailty.

## CHSP (Commonwealth Home Support Programme)

Entry-level government funding that supports older people to remain living at home. Services may include domestic assistance, meals, transport, home maintenance and social support.

## Dementia

A general term describing a group of conditions that affect memory, thinking, behaviour and the ability to perform everyday tasks. Alzheimer's disease is the most common form of dementia.

## Enduring Power of Attorney (EPOA)

A legal document allowing a trusted person to make financial and property decisions on behalf of another person if they lose decision-making capacity.

## Enduring Guardian / Medical Decision Maker

A person legally appointed to make health and lifestyle decisions for someone who no longer has capacity. The exact title varies between Australian states and territories.

## Home Care Package (HCP)
Government funding allocated to support older people with complex needs to live safely at home. Packages fund services such as personal care, nursing, allied health and home modifications. These packages are transitioning into the new Support at Home Program.

## Hospice
A specialised facility providing end-of-life care focused on comfort and symptom management for people approaching the final stage of life.

## Means Test
An assessment used to determine whether a person must contribute to the cost of aged care services based on their income and assets.

## My Aged Care
The Australian Government's central entry point for aged care information, assessments and service referrals. Most people begin their aged care journey by contacting My Aged Care.

## Palliative Care
Specialised medical care focused on improving quality of life for people with serious illness. It aims to relieve pain, breathlessness, anxiety and other distressing symptoms.

## RAD (Refundable Accommodation Deposit)
A lump-sum payment made when entering residential aged care to cover accommodation costs. The payment is refundable when the person leaves care or passes away, subject to certain conditions.

## DAP (Daily Accommodation Payment)
An alternative to paying a lump sum accommodation deposit. Instead, the resident pays a daily fee calculated using an interest rate set by the government.

## Residential Aged Care
Accommodation and care provided in a nursing home or aged care facility for people who can no longer live safely at home.

## Respite Care
Short-term care that provides temporary relief for carers. It may occur in the home, in the community or in a residential aged care facility.

### Restrictive Practices

Actions or interventions used to control behaviour that may limit a person's freedom of movement or decision-making. These include physical restraint, chemical restraint and environmental restrictions. Strict regulations govern their use.

### RAS (Regional Assessment Service)

Assesment teams that evaluate eligibility for entry-level home support services under the Commonwealth Home Support Programme.

### Serious Incident Response Scheme (SIRS)

A national system requiring aged care providers to report and respond to serious incidents including abuse, neglect or inappropriate use of restraint.

### Support at Home Program

A major aged care reform program replacing the Home Care Package and Commonwealth Home Support Programme. It aims to simplify funding and expand support for older people living at home.

### Tribunal

A legal body in each state or territory that may appoint guardians or administrators when a person can no longer make their own decisions and no suitable legal arrangements are in place.

### Voluntary Assisted Dying (VAD)

A legal process in some Australian states that allows eligible adults with advanced and incurable illness to request medical assistance to end their life. Strict eligibility criteria and safeguards apply.

### Wellbeing Principle

A central concept in the new Aged Care Act that places the wellbeing, dignity and rights of older people at the centre of aged care services and decision-making.

www.ingramcontent.com/pod-product-compliance
Lightning Source LLC
Chambersburg PA
CBHW052033280526
45791CB00010B/2949